SPIRITUALITY IN PATIENT CARE

Harold G. Koenig, M.D.

SPIRITUALITY IN PATIENT CARE

Why, How, When, and What

REVISED & EXPANDED SECOND EDITION

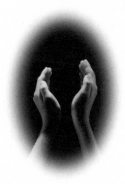

TEMPLETON FOUNDATION PRESS

Philadelphia & London

Templeton Foundation Press
300 Conshohocken State Road, Suite 670
West Conshohocken, PA 19428
www.templetonpress.org

Second edition 2007
First edition published 2002

Templeton Foundation Press helps intellectual leaders and others learn about
science research on aspects of realities, invisible and intangible. Spiritual
realities include unlimited love, accelerating creativity, worship, and the
benefits of purpose in persons and in the cosmos.

Designed and typeset by Kachergis Book Design

LIBRARY OF CONGRESS CATALOGING-IN-PUBLICATION DATA
Koenig, Harold George.
    Spirituality in patient care : why, how, when, and what / Harold G. Koenig.
— 2nd ed.
        p. ; cm.
    Includes bibliographical references and index.
    ISBN-13: 978-1-59947-116-7 (pbk. : alk. paper)
    ISBN-10: 1-59947-116-7 (pbk. : alk. paper)   1. Medical care.
2. Spirituality.   I. Title. [DNLM: 1. Spirituality.   2. Pastoral Care.
3. Patient Care—methods.   4. Patient Care—psychology.   5. Religion and
Medicine. WM 61 K78s 2007]
    R725.55.K64 2007
    615.8'52—dc22
                                                    2007002321
Printed in the United States of America

07   08   09   10   11   12   10 9 8 7 6 5 4 3 2 1

To my son, Jordan Taylor Koenig,
and my daughter, Rebekah Marie Koenig

CONTENTS

SPIRITUALITY IN PATIENT CARE

INTRODUCTION

Similar to the first edition, this volume provides a short course for health professionals (HPs) interested in identifying and addressing the spiritual needs of patients. Since the first edition, written in 2001 and published in 2002, more research has been done on the relationship between religion, spirituality and health, and further discussions have occurred on the sensible application of findings to clinical practice. In studying this research literature and interacting with literally hundreds of groups of HPs (physicians, nurses, chaplains, pastoral counselors, social workers, psychologists, counselors, physical and occupational therapists, administrators) and community clergy over the past five years, I have learned a great deal more about the religion-health care connection. HPs have also told me the areas that they felt most uncomfortable about and needed additional information on.

Therefore, I have rewritten and updated all sections of the first edition to provide the most recent research and current views on integrating spirituality into patient care. Since the *Handbook of Religion and Health*[1] was published in 2001, literally thousands of discussions, reviews, and research studies have been published, contributing new information that has advanced our understanding and provided more complete guidance. An online search of articles using the keywords "spirituality," "religion," "religiousness," or "religiosity" yielded over five thousand research articles, reviews, and discussions from 2001 to 2005.[2] Although this figure is affected by the inclusion of pastoral care journals in online databases since 2000, they account for only a relatively small proportion of these articles. Since the online search was completed in early 2006, there have been hundreds more such publications.

In addition to updating the information presented in the first edition, this second edition of *Spirituality in Patient Care* includes new sections that make this book relevant not only to physicians in primary care and the medical and surgical specialties, but also to psychiatrists and other mental health professionals, nurses, chaplains, pastoral counselors, social workers, and occupational and physical therapists. Furthermore, this new edition includes important health care information related to specific religious traditions that HPs are likely to encounter, as well as a model educational curriculum that can be used in medical schools and other HP training programs with only a few minor adaptations for each setting.

Is there need for such a guide today? Consider these facts. The Joint Commission for the Accreditation of Hospital Organizations (JCAHO) requires that a spiritual history be taken on every patient admitted to an acute care hospital or a nursing home, or seen by a home health agency, and that spiritual history must be documented in the medical record.[3] The latest edition of *Fundamentals of Nursing* has over twenty references to spirituality in the index.[4] The North American Nursing Diagnosis Association's *Nursing Diagnoses,*[5] *Nursing Interventions Classification,*[6] and *Nursing Outcome Classification*[7] each contain very specific references to spiritual diagnosis, interventions, and outcomes. Likewise, the American Association of Medical Colleges has endorsed the need to train medical students to "incorporate awareness of spirituality, and culture beliefs and practices, into the care of patients in a variety of clinical contexts . . . [and to] recognize that their own spirituality, and cultural beliefs and practices, might affect the ways they relate to, and provide care to, patients."[8] Over 100 of the 141 American medical schools now have elective or required courses on religion, spirituality, and medicine, including such places as Johns Hopkins, Harvard, and Stanford.[9]

Despite this, however, few HPs today inquire about the spiritual needs of patients. In the United States, only about 10 percent of physicians often or always take a spiritual history, and nearly 50 percent never take one.[10] The situation does not improve much among seriously ill or dying patients; even in religious areas of the country, only about 7 percent of such patients have a spiritual history documented in their medical records by a physician.[11] Many nurses also do not address these issues, despite the fact that nursing has its historical roots in the religious professions. (Until the turn of the twentieth century, virtually all nursing care was done by religious orders, and in the United Kingdom, competency in assessing the spiritual needs of patients remains a requirement for registration.)[12] The percentage of nurses who take a spiritual history is currently unknown (a task that often falls on nurses because of the JCAHO requirement), and by spiritual history I don't mean simply recording the denomination or asking if the patient wants to see a chaplain. It is safe to say that nurses today often do not take the kind of spiritual history that would fulfill even the minimum JCAHO requirement[13] (see chapter 8 for related research). Given that over three-quarters of patients report spiritual or religious needs during hospitalization,[14] an important question is, who in the hospital setting is identifying and addressing these needs?

When HPs are asked about the barriers to communicating with patients about these issues, a common response is that there are others both within and outside the health care system available to do this (chaplains and community clergy), so health care professionals don't need to. But is that true? Although community clergy often go to heroic extremes to see members of their congregation when they are acutely hospitalized, living in nursing homes, or when homebound,[15] most clergy are not trained to deal with the complex spiritual needs that occur during acute medical or chronic disabling illness. Furthermore, they often don't have the time to do so. There are many other priorities that pull on the sleeves of today's pastors, rabbis, imams, and priests, and the time pressures they face are not that much different from those that physicians and nurses encounter. Furthermore, many patients may not be regular churchgoers and won't have clergy to visit them, and many seriously ill patients will be receiving care at a location far from their local church.

Chaplains receive extensive training to address the spiritual needs of medical patients. However, under intense pressure to reduce the costs of services, hospitals have been reducing their pastoral care services or combining them with social services. In a study of 370 randomly sampled pastoral care departments, now over seven years old, 27 percent of department directors reported budgetary cutbacks.[16] And the situation appears to be growing worse. Over fifteen years ago, all full-time chaplain positions in

Georgia's state psychiatric hospitals were eliminated to help make up for the state's budget deficit,[17] and this situation remains the same today, according to my recent conversation with Gary Batchelor, a chaplain in Rome, Georgia. In the past few years, other hospitals have completely removed chaplain services to contain costs (for example, the 541-bed Hahnemann University Hospital in Philadelphia). The result is that even in acute care hospitals, there are not enough chaplains to see every patient and family and meet the needs of hospital staff. In fact, studies indicate that only about 20 percent (ranging from 10% to 30%) of acutely hospitalized patients in the United States see a chaplain.[18] Furthermore, most nursing homes have no chaplains on staff, nor are chaplains readily available in outpatient medical or psychiatric settings.

If clergy and chaplains are not able to evaluate most patients, then someone needs to. Non-chaplain HPs can assist by briefly assessing every patient to learn about religious or spiritual beliefs that might influence medical care, identify spiritual needs that could interfere with recovery from illness, and refer those patients with spiritual needs to chaplains or to other pastoral care experts. Which HP should be responsible for this screening (i.e., taking a brief spiritual history)?

There are numerous reasons why the physician, as head of the health care team, should take responsibility for initiating this dialogue with patients and for identifying spiritual needs that require further attention. Since all patients need such screening, and a lot of this information relates to medical care and medical decisions, the physician is ideally positioned to conduct a spiritual history during a hospital admission or a new evaluation of a severely or chronically ill patient. If the physician fails to carry out this task, which now is the case for 90 percent of physicians, then it naturally falls to the nurse. If the nurse fails, then the social worker or other allied health professional who sees the patient regularly must do it. Bear in mind that non-chaplain HPs are only being asked to do a brief *screening* evaluation, not a comprehensive assessment that the trained health care chaplain might do if issues came up during the HP evaluation, prompting referral.[19] Because most hospitals today are not even meeting the minimal requirements for a spiritual history established by JCAHO, it is not surprising that patient satisfaction surveys by organizations such as Press Ganey find that the meeting of emotional and spiritual needs during hospitalization is among the lowest ranked of all clinical care indicators and highest in need of quality improvement.[20]

There is a long list of reasons why HPs say they do not take a spiritual history. They don't feel comfortable talking with patients about the subject; they don't understand why they should be responsible for collecting this information; they don't know how or when to take a spiritual history, are afraid of how much time it will take, don't know what to do with the information obtained, and don't know how to respond to patients' questions that may come up. In other words, they lack the necessary training, don't feel religion/spirituality falls into their area of expertise, and are confused about what is expected of them. That is why this book is necessary.

Addressing spiritual issues in patient care is an extension of patient-centered medicine.[21] Here I address the why's, how's, when's, and what's of doing so. At a very minimum, this book will provide HPs with the training necessary to sensitively and competently screen patients for spiritual needs, to begin to communicate with patients about these issues, and to learn when to refer patients to trained spiritual care professionals who can competently address spiritual needs.

Why? Why should HPs be aware of and prepared to assess spir-

itual issues as part of routine patient care? I examine six reasons why in chapter 1: (1) many patients wish HPs to be aware
of their religious or spiritual backgrounds; (2) religious beliefs are
common among patients and help them to cope; (3) hospitalized
patients are often isolated from their religious communities and
alternative means of addressing spiritual needs should be provided; (4) religious beliefs can influence medical decisions, may
sometimes conflict with medical care, and can influence the HP-
patient relationship (affecting compliance); (5) religious beliefs
and practices often impact mental and physical health outcomes
in one way or another; and (6) religious involvement may affect
the kind of support and care patients receive in the community.
These six reasons underscore the need for HP training in this area.
The chapter concludes by a review of how physicians feel about
addressing spiritual issues and what they are currently doing.

How? How does a non-chaplain HP integrate spirituality into
patient care? What exactly is "spirituality"? In chapter 2, I go into
the specifics of taking a screening spiritual history. I review what
information is most necessary to collect. I present several different
assessment tools for taking a spiritual history, indicate the clinical setting they are best used in, and point out strengths of each
tool. I then discuss sensible interventions that HPs can do and
how to go about this, including orchestrating resources, supporting patients' spiritual beliefs, referring to pastoral services, and, if
certain stringent conditions are met, praying with patients. I also
discuss how and where this information should be documented
(to avoid duplication of effort and irritating patients).

When? In chapter 3, I address a number of important issues
with regard to the *timing* of the spiritual history and spiritual interventions. When is the spiritual history taken during the course of
the medical evaluation—as part of the chief complaint, history of

the present illness, family history, social history, physical exam, wrap-up, or as a stand-alone evaluation separate from the traditional medical history? Are certain kinds of patients and settings more appropriate than others (for example, a teenager being seen for a wart removal, a pregnant woman having a prenatal exam, an older person seen for a health maintenance visit, or someone admitted to a hospital, nursing home, or hospice)? How often should a spiritual history be taken: once and never repeated, at every visit, or only at select times? When is prayer with patients appropriate and what conditions must be met before this is permissible? When is referral to pastoral care necessary?

What? What are the benefits of taking a spiritual history? What results can be expected from assessing patients' spiritual needs? Based on recent research, chapter 4 discusses the impact that a brief spiritual history can have on the patient's ability to cope with illness, on the doctor-patient relationship, on patient compliance, and, more broadly, on the course of medical illness and response to treatment. Both positive and negative consequences are discussed, including benefits to health professionals. Uncomfortable clinical situations that may result when HPs address spiritual issues are discussed, and appropriate ways to respond are illustrated.

Boundaries and Barriers. In chapter 5, I explore limits in what the non-chaplain HP can do in this area. The kinds of questions addressed here involve boundary concerns, areas of expertise, and problems that may result if attention is not paid to such issues. Are there ethical boundaries that HPs should not cross? Does an HP's specialty make a difference? Are there gray areas that must be addressed on a case-by-case basis? What kinds of pitfalls and dangers can arise when HPs go beyond simple assessment and attempt to address spiritual needs or implement more advanced spiritual interventions? How can these problems be avoided? What are some of the resistances, fears, and concerns that prevent HPs from addressing religious/spiritual issues?

When Religion (or Spirituality) Is Harmful. No doubt, religion can have negative effects, and I discuss these in chapter 6. Are there times when religious beliefs can actually interfere with medical care, lead to health problems, or worsen disease outcomes? How can HPs handle these cases in a sensitive, thoughtful, and effective manner? Much has been said about religion causing harm, but what about "spirituality"? Can spirituality, a term that is more politically correct today than "religion," cause harm? Are there circumstances when inquiring about religious or spiritual topics or intervening in these areas can increase patient anxiety, induce guilt, or otherwise adversely affect the patient? What are some examples and how often does this occur?

Chaplains and Pastoral Care. Professional chaplains are the only HPs trained to address the spiritual needs of patients, and their unique qualifications and position within the health care system distinguish them from other HPs and from community clergy and establish them as specialized consultants. In fact, the World Health Organization has pastoral intervention codes in some versions of the International Classification of Diseases (ICD-10) (assessment-96186, ministry-96187, counseling/education-96087, ritual/worship-96109).[22] The training that certified chaplains receive is equivalent to or surpasses the amount of time that many other HPs spend on certification. In chapter 7, I discuss the role of the chaplain, pastoral counselor, and community clergy in comprehensively assessing and addressing the spiritual needs of patients. I also examine their role in meeting the emotional and spiritual needs of hospital staff, and other hospital duties that chaplains perform. Finally, I explore the overlap between what HPs are being asked to do, what chaplains and pastoral counselors are trained to do, and what community clergy can do in identifying and addressing patients' spiritual needs during hospitalization and after discharge.

Spirituality in Nursing Care. Nurses play a critical role in identifying patients' spiritual needs during hospitalization. Bedside care of the sick was the job of women religious up until the twentieth century, and many aspects of nursing care continued to have a religious emphasis until the past fifty to seventy-five years, when nursing became professionalized and scientific. However, assessing and addressing spiritual needs would seem to be a natural part of the job of nurses, given that the profession of nursing evolved from religious orders. These spiritual roots, however, were almost entirely lost in the past generation. Only recently has there been a resurgence of interest in and research on spirituality by nurses, including clinical interventions at the bedside (i.e., prayer, compassionate caring) or in the community (i.e., parish nursing). In chapter 8, I will briefly discuss what nurses should do in terms of addressing the spiritual needs of patients, and provide resources for those wanting more in-depth information in this area. Relationships between nurses and chaplains are also examined.

Spirituality in Social Work. Many social workers are interested in ensuring that the spiritual needs of patients and families are identified and addressed. As I have given talks to HPs around the country, I have noticed an increasing number of social workers attending these presentations. Chapter 9 discusses the role of medical social workers in identifying spiritual issues among patients and families and in ensuring that spiritual needs identified during hospitalization are addressed when patients return home (or are discharged to nursing homes). Community social workers can also play an important role in identifying and addressing spiritual needs of patients who are relocating to a different living situation, and this too is discussed.

Spirituality in Rehabilitation. When patients undergo the strenuous, demanding, and often painful process of rehabilitating after an injury, accident, stroke, or surgical operation, spiritual factors can play a major role in maintaining motivation and hope. Physical and occupational therapists have seen this in their patients and so have considerable interest in addressing spiritual issues. National and international membership societies now exist to help rehabilitation specialists integrate spirituality into their work as well as develop and maintain their own spirituality. Chapter 10 covers material that will be informative for specialists in this area based on systematic research by therapists themselves.

Spirituality in Mental Health Care. Chapter 11 specifically addresses what mental health professionals can do to integrate spirituality into the care of patients with psychiatric illness. Information on mental health services delivered by clergy is examined, and conflicts between mental health providers and religious professionals are discussed. Important questions explored include the following: What does a psychiatric spiritual history consist of? How do therapists address spiritual issues that come up in psychotherapy? Are spiritual interventions in this area the same or different from spiritual interventions in nonpsychiatric patients? Are there special issues related to boundaries that must be more carefully negotiated by mental health professionals than by medical care providers?

A Model Course Curriculum. Medical, nursing, social work, and rehabilitation training programs are now including elective or required courses on religion, spirituality, and health care. Currently, there is no widely used medical curriculum for physicians on how to integrate spirituality into patient care, nor is there any commonly used curriculum for other HPs either. This lack of agreement on what should be taught to HPs is a serious impediment to the field. To address this lack, chapter 12 outlines a basic ten-session model curriculum for courses on religion, spirituality, and medicine that covers most of the material in this book. I also describe how this basic curriculum can be adapted for the training of nurses, social workers, and rehabilitation specialists.

Information on Specific Religions. In an increasingly pluralistic society, HPs must take care of patients from many different religious traditions (or no tradition), and these traditions often have specific rules on health care practices that surround birth, diet, sickness, and death. For the Orthodox Jew, the devout Muslim, or the Hindu believer, there are specific rituals that must be attended to. HPs need a concise source of information about health-related sacred traditions for each major religious group, and chapter 13 has been added to meet that need.

Finally, chapter 14 provides a concise summary of the most important points the HP should be aware of when attempting to integrate spirituality into patient care. It includes the sixteen key concepts that readers of this book will want to come away with and teach to their students. These pages can be photocopied and handed out as a concise summary of what HPs need to know.

Although this book will not provide the HP with everything he or she will ever need to know about competently addressing religious or spiritual issues in patient care, it is a good place to start and will point the reader to resources that will further develop skills in this area.

CHAPTER 1

WHY INCLUDE SPIRITUALITY?

Why include spirituality in patient care? Why would an HP take time to address spiritual needs or support a patient's religious beliefs? HPs need to be able to answer such questions clearly and unambiguously before deciding to tackle spiritual issues with patients. Here are six reasons why HPs should do so:

1. Many patients are religious or spiritual, and would like it addressed in their health care.

2. Religion influences the patient's ability to cope with illness.

3. Patients, particularly when hospitalized, are often isolated from their religious communities.

4. Religious beliefs affect medical decisions and may conflict with medical treatments.

5. Religious involvement is associated with both mental and physical health, and likely affects health outcomes (one way or another).

6. Religion influences health care in the community.

MANY PATIENTS ARE RELIGIOUS

Many patients in American health care settings are religious and have spiritual needs. According to a 1996 Gallup survey, 96 percent of Americans believe in God, over 90 percent pray, nearly 70 percent are church members, and over 40 percent have attended church, synagogue, or temple within the past seven days.[1] Similarly, a September 2006 Gallup poll found that 57 percent of Americans indicated that religion was very important to them, and that figure increased to 72 percent for Americans over age sixty-five.[2] Even if patients are not religious, there is a good chance that some will describe themselves as spiritual, since about one in five Americans considers themselves "spiritual but not religious."[3] This is less true for older adults, who tend to be more traditionally religious and equate spirituality with religion. A 2004 study of 838 medical inpatients aged sixty or over found that 88 percent indicated that they were both religious and spiritual, 7 percent that they were spiritual but not religious, and 3 percent that they were religious but not spiritual. Only 3 percent of patients indicated they were neither religious nor spiritual.[4]

Not only are the vast majority of patients religious, but many of these religious patients have spiritual needs and would like those addressed in their health care. Being spiritual is part of who many people are—it forms the root of their identity as human beings and gives life meaning and purpose. Spiritual needs become particularly pressing at times when medical illness threatens life or way of life. In studying 101 psychiatric and medical/surgical inpatients at a Chicago hospital, investigators found that the vast majority of psychiatric patients (88%) and medical/surgical patients (76%) reported three or more religious needs during hospitalization.[5] Neglecting the spiritual dimension is just like ignoring a patient's social environment or psychological state, and results in failure to treat the "whole person."

Most of the available data on patients' attitudes toward HPs addressing spiritual needs is on physicians (little data currently exists for other HPs, and that is summarized in chapters 8–10). Studying 203 family practice inpatients in two hospitals located in the eastern United States, King and Bushwick report that about three-quarters (77%) said that physicians should consider their spiritual needs and 37 percent wanted their physicians to discuss their religious beliefs more.[6] According to other studies, between 33 percent and 84 percent of patients believe that physicians should ask about their religious or spiritual beliefs, depending on (1) the setting and severity of illness (routine office visit vs. acute hospitalization vs. terminal illness); (2) the particular religion of the patient; and (3) how religious the patient is.[7]

In a survey of medical outpatients, investigators surveyed 380 patients receiving care in family medicine clinics located in central Texas and south-central North Carolina.[8] Of those surveyed, 73 percent believed that patients should share their religious beliefs with doctors. In a study of 90 medical HIV-positive inpatients on the HIV/AIDS floor of the Yale–New Haven Hospital in Connecticut, the majority (53%) believed that it was important for patients to discuss spiritual needs with their physicians.[9] In the only survey to date involving a random sample of Americans, *USA Weekend* magazine conducted a nationwide poll of the attitudes of one thousand adults.[10] They asked whether Americans believed doctors ought to talk to patients about spiritual faith. Nearly two-thirds (63%) indicated that doctors should. This opinion increased slightly, to 67 percent, among older persons (those aged fifty-five to sixty-four).

Interestingly, 66 to 81 percent of patients say they would have greater trust in their physician if he or she asked about their religious/spiritual beliefs,[11] and other research has shown a significant improvement in the doctor-patient relationship when the physician does so.[12] Part of the rational for such inquiries is that for a significant proportion of patients (45–73%), religious beliefs are likely to influence their medical decisions when seriously ill (see below).[13]

Patients' feelings about praying with their physicians likewise range widely from 19 percent to 78 percent being in favor, depending on the setting, severity of their illness, and religiousness of the patient.[14] For example, in the Yale study of HIV/AIDS patients, 46 percent indicated that it would be helpful to have an opportunity to pray with their physicians.[15] In general, patients who are sicker and more religious want their HPs to pray with them. However, only 10–20 percent of patients report that their physicians ever asked them about spiritual issues or prayed with them.[16]

Although many patients want HPs to know about their religious or spiritual beliefs, a sizeable proportion of patients (from one-quarter to one-half) don't want to discuss these matters with physicians. When non-patients were surveyed in one study, over two-thirds when seriously ill would want to discuss their spiritual concerns with someone.[17] Most, however, wanted to discuss them with their ministers, not with their physicians. Unfortunately, ministers may not be available in medical settings when patients need to discuss these issues. Also, "discussing" religious beliefs with physicians is not the same as the physician or other HP inquiring about such beliefs, which other research suggests that many more patients are receptive to. Of course, most patients do not want HPs inquiring or discussing spiritual matters until after they have competently dealt with medical issues.[18]

MANY PATIENTS DEPEND ON RELIGION TO COPE

Not only is religion vital to the identities of many people, it is often used to cope with troubling life circumstances. According to a national Gallup survey, nearly 80 percent of Americans say that the statement "I receive a great deal of comfort and support from my religious beliefs" is completely or mostly true (especially persons over age sixty-five, 87% of whom give this response).[19] A random survey of the U.S. population one week after the terrorist attacks on September 11, 2001, published in the *New England Journal of Medicine*, found that 90 percent of Americans turned to religion in order to cope with the stress of these events.[20] Likewise, in certain parts of the United States, over 90 percent of medical patients report that religious beliefs and practices are ways that they cope with and make sense of physical illness, and over 40 percent indicate that religion is *the most important* factor that keeps them going.[21] Research shows that religious coping is widespread in patients with chronic illnesses such as heart disease,[22] arthritis,[23] kidney disease,[24] cystic fibrosis,[25] diabetes,[26] cancer,[27] gynecologic cancer,[28] HIV/AIDS,[29] chronic pain,[30] and terminal illness,[31] and in nursing home patients[32] and dementia caregivers.[33]

What exactly is "religious coping"? Religious coping is the use of religious beliefs or practices to reduce the emotional distress caused by loss or change. Patients may "turn over" their problems to God, trusting God to handle them so that they don't have to ruminate or worry about them. They may believe that God has a purpose in allowing them to experience pain or suffering, which gives suffering meaning and makes it more bearable. A host of religious cognitions like these are mobilized to reduce anxiety, increase hope, or convey a sense of control. With regard to religious practices that facilitate coping, patients may pray, meditate, read religious scriptures, attend religious services, perform religious rituals (receive the sacraments or anointing with oil, for example), or rely on support from clergy or members of their church, synagogue, mosque, or temple. Religious beliefs and practices, then, are used to *regulate emotion* during times of illness, change, and circumstances that are out of patients' personal control.

ISOLATED FROM RELIGIOUS COMMUNITIES

When patients are hospitalized in acute care, rehabilitation, or long-term care settings, they are often isolated from their religious communities. Even if they would want to discuss their spiritual concerns with their minister, ministers are often not available. HIPAA[34] regulations may even prevent clergy and religious communities from knowing whether one of their members is hospitalized. Therefore, patients may not have the ability to access their usual religious resources, as they would if they were independent, living at home, and able to travel. Furthermore, spiritual needs that arise when people become sick, disabled, or face prospects of death and dying are not easily addressed by community clergy unless they have specific training on how to do so and are connected to the HPs who are providing the health care. For these reasons, it is imperative that health care settings provide a mechanism by which patients' spiritual needs can be identified, spiritual resources provided, and referral made to pastoral care professionals adequately trained to address spiritual needs and the emotional or health-related conflicts that may arise from them. More about patient isolation will be discussed in chapter 7 on chaplains and pastoral care.

RELIGIOUS BELIEFS INFLUENCE MEDICAL DECISIONS

Religious beliefs influence the medical decisions patients make when seriously ill, and may conflict with medical treatments planned for the patient. For example, a recent study of 177 consecutive outpatients seen in the pulmonary clinic at the Hospital of the University of Pennsylvania found that nearly half of the patients (45%) indicated that religious beliefs would influence their medical decisions if they became gravely ill.[35] Religious or spiritual beliefs may also influence the medical decisions of patients with religious beliefs that are not traditional. For example, a recent study of 458 "neo-pagans" (Wiccans, Druids, Asatruans) reported that 73 percent had religious or spiritual beliefs that would influence their medical decisions.[36]

End-of-life decisions are often influenced by the religious beliefs of patients or family members, especially do-not-resuscitate or discontinuation-of-treatment decisions.[37] For example, a patient or family member may be praying for a miracle in a medically futile situation. This belief could keep hope alive and prevent them from "giving up" (even when giving up is the most appropriate thing to do). Agreeing to a no code status or foregoing aggressive therapy may mean "giving up" to the patient or family.

Religious beliefs influence other treatment decisions when the threat of death is imminent, an effect that physicians often underestimate. For example, a study of 100 patients with advanced lung cancer, their caregivers, and 257 medical oncologists attending an annual meeting of the American Society of Clinical Oncology asked participants to rank the importance of seven factors that might influence treatment decisions on whether or not to accept chemotherapy.[38] These factors included the oncologist's recommendation, faith in God, ability of treatment to cure the disease, side effects of the chemotherapy, family doctor's recommendation, spouse's recommendation, and children's recommendation. Patients, family, and physicians each ranked these factors from 1 (most important) to 7 (least important). Although patients and family members both ranked "faith in God" as 2 (outranked only by the recommendation of the oncologist), oncologists ranked faith in God last (7).

Religious beliefs can also influence the patient's diet, both in the hospital and after he or she is discharged home; practices related to birth and birth control; and rituals surrounding illness, death and dying (see chapter 13). Beliefs can influence whether patients will comply with medical treatments, accept blood, vaccinate their children, receive prenatal care, take antibiotics and other prescribed drugs, alter lifestyles, accept referral to a psychologist or psychiatrist, or even come back for medical follow-up. Unless HPs know about the patient's religious and/or spiritual beliefs, how can they adequately manage the patient's illness?

RELIGION'S RELATIONSHIP TO HEALTH

During the twentieth century, more than twelve hundred studies examined the relationship between religion and health, with the majority finding a significant positive association.[39] Many of these were cross-sectional studies and weak in terms of methodology, often because they were done without research funding, which has become available only in recent years. There were also, however, many well-designed prospective studies, and even a handful of clinical trials that verified and supported the findings from cross-sectional studies. Since the turn of the twenty-first century, many new research reports have now been published replicating and reaffirming results from earlier, less well-designed studies. Much of this research has been in areas that are relevant to patient care.

Religious Coping and Depression. Medically ill patients who rely on religion to cope adapt more quickly to illness than those who do not.[40] Patients who depend on religion are less likely to develop depression,[41] and even if they do become depressed, are more likely to recover quickly from depression than patients who are less religious.[42] This is also true for the caregivers of patients with Alzheimer's disease or cancer, who appeared to adapt more quickly to the caregiver role if more religious.[43]

Many studies in different populations have identified inverse correlations between religiousness and depression. More than a hundred studies examined this relationship during the twentieth century, including twenty-two prospective cohort studies and eight clinical trials.[44] Approximately two-thirds (65%) of observational studies found significantly lower rates of depressive disorder or fewer depressive symptoms in those who were more religious, and 68 percent of prospective studies found that greater religiousness predicted less depression. Five of the eight clinical trials reported that depressed patients who received religious interventions recovered more quickly than subjects receiving either a secular intervention or usual care.

Suicide and Substance Abuse. There is even more consensus when rates of suicide and substance abuse are considered. Of 68 studies examining suicide, 84 percent found lower rates of suicide or more negative attitudes toward it among the more religious. Of the nearly 140 studies that have examined religious involvement and abuse of alcohol or drugs, 90 percent found a statistically significant inverse correlation between the two.[45] The consistency of findings across these studies is impressive, given that they were carried out in many different populations, by different research groups, and in different areas of the world.

Positive Emotions. Well-being and positive emotions such as joy, hope, and optimism also appear to be disproportionately prevalent among the religious. Of one hundred studies in the past century that examined these relationships, seventy-nine found that religious persons had significantly greater well-being, life satisfaction, or happiness than did those who were less religious. Of sixteen studies that examined the association between religion and purpose or meaning in life, fifteen found that religious persons had significantly greater purpose and meaning in life. Even arch-enemy of religion Sigmund Freud admitted that "only religion can answer the question of the purpose of life. One can hardly be wrong in concluding that the idea of life having a purpose stands and falls with the religious system."[46]

Social Support. Almost all studies examining religion and social support find a significant correlation (19 of 20 studies).[47] Not only does the religious person have a larger support network, but the quality of that social network is higher and may be more durable than secular sources of support when chronic illness strikes.[48]

Physical Health. There is mounting evidence from the field of psychoneuroimmunology and even genetics that negative emotions and social isolation are associated with worse immune functioning and poorer cardiovascular health.[49] Perceived psychological stress may even influence the speed of cellular aging. One recent study compared stressed women to those who were less stressed, finding that the cells of stressed women were aging ten years more rapidly (based on telomere shortening with each DNA replication).[50] If religious involvement is associated with greater well-being, more social support, better coping, less depression, and lower perceived stress, then religious activities may also lead to better physical health, greater longevity, and may even affect the aging process.

Although research examining the relationship between religious involvement and immune function is only in its infancy, several published studies and other unpublished reports suggest a connection, and one that has clinical consequences. In a study of more than 1,700 randomly sampled community-dwelling older adults, we found that high levels of the cytokine interleukin-6 (IL-6) were significantly more common in those who did not attend religious services than in those who did.[51] Not long ago, the findings from this study were replicated in a different area of the country by a different research group; again, frequent church attenders had lower IL-6 levels and greater longevity (which was explained by the lower IL-6 levels).[52] IL-6 is an inflammatory indicator and levels are high in diseases like AIDS, lymphoma, and other immune disorders. IL-6 also increases with age as the immune system begins to weaken.

Not surprisingly, in light of the IL-6 studies above, a report on 112 patients with metastatic breast cancer indicated that women who scored higher on religious expression had significantly higher natural killer cell numbers, T-helper cell counts, and total lymphocytes.[53] Likewise, in a study of 106 HIV-positive homosexual men, those who were more religiously involved had significantly higher CD4+ counts and CD4+ percentages compared to those who were less religious.[54]

Most recently, a study of one hundred HIV-positive patients followed over four years found that those who reported an increase in spirituality/religiousness (S/R) after HIV diagnosis had significantly greater preservation of CD4+ cells and significantly better control of viral load during the ensuing four years.[55] Likewise, frequent church attenders at baseline also had significantly greater preservation of CD4+ cells over time. Results for increased S/R in predicting disease course were independent of church attendance and initial disease status, medications taken to control the disease, age, gender, race, education, health behaviors, depression, hopelessness, optimism coping, and social support. In fact, the size of the effects of increased S/R on CD4+ cell preservation and viral load were larger than for any other predictor.

Stress hormone levels also appear to be related to degree of religious involvement. One study found that long-term survivors with AIDS were more religious, and their greater longevity was explained by lower cortisol levels (presumably due to lower stress levels).[56] A Yale University study of women with fibromyalgia also found that cortisol rhythms were healthier among women who were more religious.[57]

With regard to cardiovascular health, at least twenty-three studies have examined the relationship between religiousness and blood pressure.[58] Over 60 percent (14 of the 23) reported lower blood pressure among the more religious. This is especially true for diastolic blood pressures, and may help to explain scattered reports of lower stroke rate[59] and lower death rate from coronary artery disease[60] among the more religious.

In fact, there is a consistent relationship between degree of religious involvement and lower mortality in general. Of fifty-two studies published before the year 2000 that examined the relationship between religiousness and mortality, 75 percent ($n=39$) found that religiously active persons lived longer than the less religious, 19 percent ($n=10$) found no difference, 4 percent ($n=2$) reported mixed results (longer or shorter, depending on type of religious activity), and 2 percent ($n=1$) found shorter survival among the more religious.[61] A metanalysis of these studies found that religiousness predicted a 29 percent increase in survival during follow-up (OR=1.29, 95% CI 1.20–1.39).[62]

These findings are particularly consistent when religiousness is measured in terms of religious community involvement. According to a random U.S. national sample of over twenty thousand adults followed for an average of eight years, the difference in survival between those who attended religious services more than weekly and those who did not attend was approximately seven years (14 years in African Americans).[63] Stated differently, religious attendance has nearly the same association with longer survival as not smoking cigarettes, especially among women.[64] Bear in mind that most of these studies control for baseline physical health and explanatory factors such as mental health, social support, and health behaviors. Even after controlling for factors thought to explain this relationship, a significant survival advantage continues to be present for the more religious.[65] Many of the more recent prospective studies that have used advanced research methods such as structural equation modeling and hierarchical linear modeling have documented some of the strongest associations between religious involvement and health.[66]

Religious involvement also predicts changes in physical and cognitive functioning as people age. Researchers at Yale University, the University of Alabama, and the University of Texas show a slowing in the decline of physical functioning and reduced fear of falling with increasing age.[67] Researchers at Yale and the University of Texas also have found that cognitive functioning declines more slowly with age among those who are more religiously active.[68] Neurology researchers at Toronto's Baycrest Centre for Geriatric Care have found that religious patients with Alzheimer's disease experience a slower decline in cognition over time.[69] Survival after major cardiac surgery also appears to be better[70] and complications fewer[71] among the more religious.

Religious or spiritual struggles may also impact health outcomes, but in a negative way. For example, when patients become sick and pray for help, and the illness continues and progresses despite these supplications, they may begin to ask, "Why me?" Spiritual struggles of this nature may include feeling that God is punishing them, God (or their faith community) has deserted them, God is unable to help, and so forth. These spiritual struggles, while normal and expected in those with diseases that cause severe suffering and life changes, can influence the course of illness unless patients are able to resolve such feelings. We followed 444 systematically identified medically ill hospitalized patients over a period of two years after discharge, assessing their level of religious struggle.[72] Those with struggles and questions like those above during the baseline hospital evaluation were significantly more likely to die during follow-up. For every one-point increase on a religious struggles scale (range 0 to 21), mortality rate increased by 6 percent. This was statistically significant and independent of physical health, social support, or mental health. Patients with religious struggles may not feel comfortable talking with a member of the clergy about such concerns because they feel angry at God or alienated from religion. However, they may broach this subject with an HP unconnected to religion, whom they see as more objective and less judgmental.

Religious beliefs may also influence decisions on whether to seek health care and whether to comply with medical treatments. Certain fatalistic beliefs such as "it's God's will" or "it's Allah's will" or "it's my karma" can and do influence patients' actions.[73] Fatalism is defined as a belief that disease is inevitable and that no medical care or personal changes can forestall death. Identifying religious struggles and fatalistic religious beliefs that affect the seeking of and compliance with medical care is one of the best reasons why HPs need to take a spiritual history.

Need for Health Services. Research suggests that religious persons spend less time in the hospital, perhaps because they are healthier and have more support within the community. In a study of 542 patients (age sixty or over) consecutively admitted to Duke University Medical Center, those who attended religious services once a week or more were 56 percent less likely to have been hospitalized during the previous year (p < .0001).[74] This finding remained significant after controlling for severity of medical illness, level of physical functioning, social support, depressive symptoms, age, sex, race, and education. In terms of actual number of days hospitalized, patients attending religious services at least several times per month were hospitalized an average of six days in the previous year, compared to twelve days for those attending services only a few times per year or not at all.

In the prospective part of the study, patients who indicated they were not affiliated with a religious group were hospitalized at Duke for an average of twenty-five days, compared to only eleven days for persons affiliated with any religious tradition. This large difference in length of stay between affiliated and non-affiliated patients could not be explained by severity of physical illness, disability level, social support, or depressive symptoms. In fact, when these other variables were controlled, the strength of the relationship between lack of religious affiliation and longer hospital stay actually became stronger. Need for long-term care services is also lower among those who are more religious, especially for women and for African Americans.[75]

Implications. There is growing evidence from systematic research that religious beliefs and practices are related to mental health, physical health, and need for health services. This research should help dispel the widespread notion among health professionals that religion is either unrelated to health or only characteristic of the neurotic.[76] Nevertheless, many questions remain unanswered. We know that religious or spiritual involvement does not *always* have positive effects on health, and even when it does so, the underlying biological mechanisms are not well understood. A host of new studies now being undertaken at leading universities are utilizing a variety of research methods, from observational designs to randomized clinical trials, to more rigorously test the associations between religion and health. However, there is plenty of evidence to date to suggest that religion, health, and medical outcomes are related, one way or another.

RELIGION INFLUENCES HEALTH CARE IN THE COMMUNITY

As health care resources become less abundant, there is pressure on hospitals to reduce the time that patients spend in the hospital (the most expensive form of health care). Hospital stays will get shorter (a trend that is already evident today) and patients with more severe and unstable medical illnesses will be discharged back into the community earlier and earlier. Many more treatments will be done in outpatient settings, and patients will spend time recovering from illness in their homes. Thus, health care needs within the community will grow and grow rapidly as the U.S. population ages.

In the days ahead, churches and other religious organizations will need to deal with many more members with chronic illness (or recovering from acute illness) and with families trying to manage these conditions at home. Religious organizations could play a major role in early disease detection (through screening), disease prevention (through education), and direct provision of health care or respite care (through trained volunteers). For this reason, HPs need to begin communicating and collaborating with religious organizations, establishing referral networks and providing education for religious organizations to prepare them and support them in meeting the needs of patients after discharge. Thus, it is essential that the HP know something about whether the patient is a member of a religious community, what that membership means to the patient, and the resources available to the patient from this source after leaving the hospital or doctor's office.

MISCELLANEOUS ISSUES

Recognizing the need for HPs to communicate with patients about spiritual issues, JCAHO requires that a spiritual history be taken and documented on every patient admitted to a hospital, nursing home, or home health care agency. It is currently monitoring whether such information is contained in the medical record and disciplining institutions that are not doing this in an appropriate fashion. This does not mean simply asking about the patient's denomination or whether he or she wants to see a chaplain, which is largely what is being recorded in most patients' medical records in the majority of medical institutions today. JCAHO has specified the minimal requirements necessary to meet the standards of care:

> Spiritual assessment should, at a minimum, determine the patient's denomination, beliefs, and what spiritual practices are important to the patient. This information would assist in determining the impact of spirituality, if any, on the care/services being provided and will identify if any further assessment is needed. The standards require organizations to define the content and scope of spiritual

and other assessments and the qualifications of the individual(s) performing the assessment.[77]

If spirituality is found during this initial screening to be of importance to the patient, JCAHO then recommends other questions that can be asked, including:

Does the patient use prayer in [his or her] life?

How does the patient express [his or her] spirituality?

What type of spiritual/religious support does the patient desire?

What is the name of the patient's clergy, ministers, chaplains, pastor, rabbi?

What are the patient's spiritual goals?

Is there a role of church/synagogue in the patient's life?

How does [the patient's] faith help the patient cope with illness?

Meeting a JCAHO requirement, though, is not a very good reason why HPs should address spiritual issues as part of routine clinical care. Rather, the other reasons outlined above that emphasize the desires of patients, the role that spiritual factors play in coping with medical illness, the isolation of patients from their religious communities, the influence of religious beliefs on medical decisions, the effects of beliefs on health outcomes, and the support that religious organizations provide in the community are much better reasons for doing so. The overall objective here is to improve the quality of patient care, address the needs of patients as whole persons, enhance their coping with illness, and ultimately improve their medical outcomes.

CURRENT ATTITUDES AND BEHAVIORS

So how do HPs feel about all this and what are they currently doing? Most of what we know is from surveys of physicians. Physicians (1) acknowledge that spiritual well-being is an important component of health (96%),[78] (2) say that they should be aware of the patient's religious/spiritual beliefs (85%),[79] and (3) indicate that they have a right to inquire about these matters (89%).[80] However, only 31 to 76 percent of physicians feel that they should ask about patients beliefs, depending on the setting (outpatient visit vs. acute hospitalization vs. terminal care). In the largest study to date that involved a national U.S. random sample of 1,144 physicians, Curlin and colleagues found that only 55 percent said that it was usually or always appropriate for the physician to inquire about the patient's R/S beliefs (and, conversely, 45% indicated that it was usually or always inappropriate to do so).[81] When behaviors were assessed, only 10 percent of physicians indicated that they often or always inquired about R/S issues, which confirms results from regional surveys.[82] There is a remarkable gap, then, between what physicians say they should be aware of (i.e., R/S beliefs of patients), their attitude toward acquiring that information (i.e., taking a spiritual history), and their actual behavior in terms of doing so. Curlin and colleagues found that the religiousness of the physician was one of the strongest factors predicting positive attitudes toward taking a spiritual history.

Besides attitudes and practices concerning asking patients about R/S beliefs, physician behaviors related to spiritual *interventions* have also been surveyed. For all practical purposes, these interventions involve praying with patients and supporting patients' religious beliefs. We asked a random sample of 160 family physicians in Illinois if they had ever prayed with an older patient and, if so, whether they thought this had helped the patient.[83] Responses indicated that 37 percent had prayed at some time in their careers with a patient, and 89 percent of the time they indicated it benefited the patient. In that study, 88 percent of physicians felt that it was appropriate to pray with a sick older patient if the patient requested prayer.

When Monroe and colleagues asked a regional sample of 476 physicians (the majority of whom were internists and in residency training or fellowship) about the appropriateness of prayer, they found that attitudes varied depending on setting: 6 percent said that a physician should pray with a patient during a routine office visit, 14 percent if the patient is acutely hospitalized (but not near death), and 27 percent if the patient is dying. If the patient requested prayer, on the other hand, approval of physician-patient prayer increased to 56 percent during a routine office visit, 63 percent for hospitalized patients, and 77 percent for dying patients.[84]

In Curlin and colleagues' national sample of physicians, they found that 17 percent indicated it was never appropriate to pray with a patient, 55 percent indicated that it was only appropriate to pray if the patient asked, and 29 percent indicated that it was appropriate if the physician sensed that prayer was indicated (i.e., if the physician initiated the prayer).[85] In terms of behavior, they found that 19 percent of physicians sometimes, often, or always prayed with their patients, whereas 34 percent rarely and 48 percent never did so. Again, prayer with patients depended largely on the religiousness of the physician; only 30 percent of those who were low on religiousness/spirituality ever prayed with patients, whereas 76 percent of physicians high on religiousness/spirituality prayed with patients. Thus, it appears that the majority of physicians feel that prayer is most appropriate if the patient is sicker and initiates a request for prayer, although similar to taking a spiritual history, most physicians rarely or never do so unless they themselves are religious.

With regard to supporting the patient's religious beliefs, Curlin and colleagues found that 73 percent of their national sample of 1,144 physicians indicated they often or always encourage the patient's own religious/spiritual beliefs and practices, with religious physicians doing so more frequently. This is the only data, to my knowledge, on physician attitudes toward supporting patients' R/S beliefs.

Thus, many patients wish their physicians would know about their religious or spiritual beliefs, and a significant minority wishes to engage in religious activities with them. Older adults, those with more serious medical illnesses, and those who are more religious are especially likely to desire this. Some patients, however, do not wish physicians to either pray with them or inquire about their religious beliefs (especially during routine office visits), underscoring the need for sensitivity when addressing these issues. From the physician's perspective, most feel that spiritual well-being is an important part of health and therefore they should be aware of patients' R/S beliefs. However, only about half of physicians say that they should ask patients about their R/S beliefs, and only about one in ten physicians say that they regularly do so.

SUMMARY AND CONCLUSIONS

Good reasons exist for identifying and addressing the spiritual needs of patients. Many patients are religious and use religious beliefs and practices to cope with illness. Because of this, religious beliefs often influence medical decisions, especially when illness is serious or terminal. Many patients would like HPs to be aware of their spiritual needs and support them in this area. This is particularly true if they are religious, older, and their illness is serious or chronic. Furthermore, a growing research database indicates that in the majority of cases, religious beliefs and practices are related to better mental health, quality of life, and medical outcomes.

HPs addressing the spiritual needs of patients is not something new, and the history of medicine documents these practices.[86] What is new, and only within the past generation, has been the exclusion of these matters from health care. The rationale for that approach is becoming weaker and weaker in the face of growing scientific evidence supporting the religion-health connection and just plain common sense. However, sensibly reintegrating spirituality back into patient care will be a challenge, and many HPs are resistant to doing so. How one goes about addressing spiritual issues in this day and age, then, is the subject of the next chapter.

CHAPTER 2

HOW TO INCLUDE SPIRITUALITY

How does an HP include spirituality in patient care? What exactly is spirituality? How does one go about identifying spiritual needs? What does one do with the information learned? How does the HP respond to questions from the patient about this? By HP, I mean an HP without religious training (the role of the professional chaplain will be discussed in chapter 7). This chapter describes the "screening" spiritual history and provides specific recommendations on how to proceed in addressing the spiritual needs uncovered. Recommendations include, but are not limited to, listening in order to understand, showing respect for R/S beliefs, supporting the patient's spiritual beliefs, and appropriate referral. While there are boundaries that HPs should not cross and some activities that are quite controversial (praying with patients), sensible approaches are possible. Finally, this chapter explores how HPs and health care systems can link together with religious communities through parish nurses or lay leaders to address health needs in the community.

WHAT IS SPIRITUALITY?

When clinicians broach this topic with patients, it is important to use a broad definition of spirituality. The dialogue must begin somewhere, and the net should be cast as widely as possible so that all patients feel like they have a place at the table. The word "spirituality" is sufficiently broad, vague, and undefined to include almost everyone. Thus, clinicians should usually use "spiritual" terminology rather than talking about religion, which may alienate some patients. However, addressing issues in clinical practice is different from understanding what *the research* on spirituality and health really means. Therefore, I will digress for a moment to address this issue, since the assessment process and clinical applications depend to some degree on what we're talking about here—in other words, what the word "spirituality" actually means and how it's related to health.

Almost every patient, clinician, and researcher in the field of spirituality and health has his or her own definition of the term "spirituality." Some of these definitions are so broad that they include almost every human experience—from winning a basketball game, to viewing a sunset, to a sexual experience, to a deep, whole-hearted belief in and commitment to a religious tradition. Everyone is talking about something different. This lack of consensus on the very meaning of the term at the center of this discussion, while a benefit in clinical practice, is a huge impediment to research on spirituality and health. This is especially true for understanding and interpreting the research that has already been done, on which the rationale for integrating spirituality into clinical care heavily rests.

As it is currently used in research and clinical discussions today, the word "spirituality" has often been neutered of religion and transformed into a psychological construct with almost no distinctive aspects.[1] In studies claiming to measure spirituality, the actual questions tapping this construct have either been measured by religion (where religion and spirituality are synonymous), or have been assessed by questions about "peacefulness," "connectedness to others," "purpose and meaning," "feelings of wonder or awe," "forgiveness," "gratitude," "existential well-being," and other quasi-indicators of good mental health. This latter way of assessing spirituality heavily influences the research findings.

When spirituality defined as good mental health is correlated with mental health constructs such as depression, suicidal thoughts, anxiety, or other indicators of mental illness, an inverse correlation invariably results. Researchers then conclude that spirituality is related to better mental health, less mental illness, and, because mental health often affects physical health, better physical health as well. Thus, spirituality defined as good mental health is found to correlate with good mental health. Is this good research? No. It is called tautology—a circular kind of reasoning where a construct is being correlated with itself. This is a serious flaw in the spirituality and health research being carried out today. Even a cursory review of studies purporting to examine spirituality, which ought to include an examination of the questions being asked to assess spirituality, will demonstrate this point.

The diffuseness and psychological nature of the word "spirituality" as it is used today are a result of admirable attempts to be inclusive—inclusive of many different belief systems, religious and nonreligious—and to not offend or alienate anyone. And, as pointed out earlier, that is especially important for addressing spirituality in clinical practice. The result, however, is a term that has become diluted and often meaningless, centered on positive emotions and concepts. As Smith and Denton point out, "The very idea and language of 'spirituality,' originally grounded in the self-disciplining faith practices of religious believers, including ascetics and monks, then becomes detached from its moorings in historical religious traditions and is redefined in terms of subjective self-fulfillment."[2] Spirituality is more than that.

Ken Pargament defines the word "spirituality" as "a search for the sacred."[3] Pargament has been one of the leaders attempting to ground the term spirituality in something more substantial, that is, the "sacred" (God, Jesus, Mohammed, the Buddha, Brahman, ultimate truth or reality). Although not perfect, this is a major improvement over definitions commonly used today and at least gives spirituality some kind of distinctiveness (different from positive psychology), yet is still broad enough to be inclusive of persons who are either affiliated with a traditional religion or not. With these considerations in mind, let us proceed with the spiritual history.

THE SPIRITUAL HISTORY

Taking a spiritual history is the central and most important activity that HPs are being asked to do. Nothing should be done in this area, including referral to pastoral care or involvement in spiritual activity such as prayer with patients, before the spiritual history is completed. The spiritual history will determine all future interventions in this area and may impact the medical care plan being developed for the patient.

Taking a brief spiritual history is necessary in order to (1) understand the role that religion plays in the patient's coping with illness or in causing him or her stress, (2) become familiar with the patient's religious beliefs as they relate to decisions about medical care, and (3) identify patient spiritual needs that could affect health outcomes if not adequately addressed. Taking a spiritual history is a powerful act in itself and serves many purposes, in addition to those just mentioned. First, it sends a message to the patient that this aspect of his or her identity is recognized and respected by the HP. Second, it gathers important information that is useful for understanding the motivation behind many of the patient's behaviors related to health care. Third, it provides information about patients' support systems and resources within the community that can help ensure that patients comply with treatment, obtain adequate medical follow-up, and have people around them to monitor their conditions and provide necessary care. Finally, it lets the patient know that this is an area that the HP is willing to discuss in the future, should the need arise.

Several instruments have been used to take a spiritual history (see below). While it is not essential that the HP use one of these instruments, it is important that certain information be collected and done so in a sensitive manner. When choosing an instrument to take a spiritual history, then, there are five qualities that should be considered. First, the questions should be brief and take only a few minutes to administer. Brevity is a practical necessity, given the amount of other information that the HP must gather during a medical history. Second, the questions must be easy to remember so that important information is not missed. Third, the questions should be effective in gathering the type of information sought (i.e., have appropriate content for the particular situation). Fourth, the questions should focus on the patient's beliefs—the history must be patient-centered. The information being gathered has nothing whatsoever to do with the HP's beliefs. The purpose is to understand the patient's beliefs and what role they play in health and illness, without judgment or attempt to modify those beliefs or lack of belief. Finally, the instrument should have cred-ibility, that is, it must be acknowledged by experts in the field as valid and appropriate. Below are examples of three short spiritual histories that meet most of these criteria. Each has its advantages and disadvantages, and choice of instrument depends on personal preference, setting, and time available.

CSI-MEMO Spiritual History

This four-item spiritual history, originally published in the *Journal of the American Medical Association* (JAMA),[4] has been adapted for a busy clinical setting—particularly for hospitalized patients for whom a treatment plan is being developed. It inquires about four aspects of the patient's spiritual history that are immediately relevant to patient care during and after hospitalization.

1. Do your religious/spiritual beliefs provide **C**omfort, or are they a source of **S**tress?

2. Do you have spiritual beliefs that might **I**nfluence your medical decisions?

3. Are you a **MEM**ber of a religious or spiritual community, and is it supportive to you?

4. Do you have any **O**ther spiritual needs that you'd like someone to address?

This spiritual history is brief, has a credible source, and will identify most issues that could affect medical decision making or trigger a referral to a chaplain or pastoral counselor. Not all this information needs to be collected at one time, although all of it is relevant to patient care and should eventually be obtained for hospitalized patients. The mnemonic CSI-MEMO may be used to remember these questions.

ACP Spiritual History

A consensus panel of the American College of Physicians and American Society of Internal Medicine has suggested that the following four simple questions be asked of patients in palliative care, the setting in which these questions were developed.[5]

1. Is faith (religion, spirituality) important to you in this illness?
2. Has faith been important to you at other times in your life?
3. Do you have someone to talk to about religious matters?
4. Would you like to explore religious matters with someone?

This spiritual history has a credible source in a prominent medical body and has been published in a major medical journal. The instrument is brief and easy to remember. It is also patient centered and does not get too personal by having the HP offer to personally address the patient's spiritual needs. This tool was published in the *Annals of Internal Medicine* in an article authored by a trio of academic giants (Bernard Lo, a medical ethicist at the University of California at San Francisco; Timothy Quill, a highly respected and widely known physician-author; and James Tulsky, a prominent medical internist and ethicist at Duke). A major weakness, however, is that the questions fail to gather information in several key content areas (identifying spiritual needs, connections with spiritual community, and beliefs affecting medical decisions).

FICA Spiritual History

Christina Puchalski, associate professor of medicine at George Washington University Medical Center and director of the George Washington Institute for Spirituality and Health, has developed the following five questions that are easily remembered using the income tax mnemonic FICA:[6]

1. F—faith—What is your faith tradition?
2. I—important—How important is your faith to you?
3. C—church—What is your church or community of faith?
4. A—apply—How do your religious and spiritual beliefs apply to your health?
5. A—address—How might we address your spiritual needs?

This instrument is also brief, has reasonably good content, is patient centered, has been published in a peer-reviewed medical journal, and is easy to remember, meeting all five qualities needed in an assessment tool. It is ideal for conducting a spiritual history in outpatient settings.

Single Question Spiritual History

Each of the above spiritual histories takes time to administer, and will add a few minutes to the medical encounter. In clinical situations that are rushed and do not allow more than a few moments to take the spiritual history, the HP may only have time to ask one question. I suggest the following:

"Do you have any spiritual needs or concerns related to your health?"

Such a question will at least acknowledge to the patient that this is an area that the HP is concerned about and, if necessary, will open the door for any future conversation about spiritual issues.

Before beginning the spiritual history, the HP should explain to the patient why these questions are being asked. If the subject of spirituality or religion is brought up without first preparing the patient, the topic may cause undue anxiety or panic. Patients may have had experiences with other family members or friends where the only time that the doctor spoke about religion was when the patient was really sick or nothing else could be done. Patients are always looking for cues about how their conditions are progressing, and may literally hang on every word the HP says. For that reason, the HP should communicate to the patient that he or she has a few questions about spiritual beliefs, and that this has nothing to do with the patient's condition but rather reflects a desire to be more sensitive to spiritual beliefs or needs that some patients may have. After it is clear that the patient understands, the spiritual history may proceed.

It is essential that the HP collect this information in a sensitive and respectful manner. Delegating these questions to the chaplain is not sufficient, since 80 percent of patients will not see a chaplain. The HP needs to take a spiritual history in order to communicate to the patient that he or she is willing to talk about these issues if they become relevant to the patient's care. Furthermore, asking these questions will provide firsthand knowledge of the answers so that the HP can assure that spiritual needs are met and that medical decisions are made in light of them.

NONRELIGIOUS PATIENTS

What does the HP do when a patient indicates at the beginning of the spiritual history that he or she has no interest in religion or spirituality and that these factors play no role in coping with illness? As soon as the patient communicates this message to the HP, the spiritual history should take a different tack. Rather than focus on spirituality or religion, the HP might ask about how the patient is coping, what gives life meaning and purpose in the setting of the current illness (grandchildren, hobbies, etc.), what cultural beliefs are held that may influence the treatment of the illness, and what social resources are available to provide support at home. In this way, vital information is collected while not offending the patient or making the patient feel uncomfortable or pressured. This approach will allow patients to address religious or spiritual issues at their own pace, or not at all. It is especially important that the HP not make the patient feel guilty for not being religious (more will be said about this later).

More controversial is to what extent, if at all, the HP should inform nonreligious patients about spiritual resources available to them, should they wish to pursue them. Is it fair to deprive nonreligious patients of information about available spiritual resources that other patients have access to (i.e., services offered by chaplains, time when chapel services are held, prayer with HPs who are willing to do this)? If the HP provides such information, it must be done in a way that does not infringe on the free and unrestricted *choice* of the patient, and the patient's choice *not to* receive information on spiritual resources must be respected and preserved at all times.

BEYOND SCREENING

Taking a brief spiritual history will provide the HP with important information about the patient's spirituality and the patient's spiritual needs brought on by illness. What does the HP do next? Having identified spiritual needs, what is the role of the HP in documenting and addressing those needs? Almost no research has been done to help guide us in determining which actions are more or less appropriate for HPs to engage in, and there remains plenty of controversy on how much the HP should do, other than taking a brief spiritual history. In this section, I discuss the following HP activities that might follow the spiritual history: documentation, orchestrating resources (including pastoral care referral), supporting spiritual beliefs, participating in spiritual activities (such as prayer), prescribing spiritual activities, and working together with religious communities to optimize health care and ensure monitoring in the community.

Documentation. Ideally, a special section of the medical record should be designated for documenting the spiritual history, lack of spiritual interest, presence of specific spiritual needs, and any follow-up done by pastoral care. This will help avoid the problem of several HPs taking a spiritual history, duplicating each other's work, and overwhelming or irritating the patient. Any HP can simply turn to this section of the medical record to see if the spiritual history has been taken and what was learned. The introduction of the electronic medical record into clinical settings will help to make such documentation easier and faster to locate. Taking the history and documenting it in the medical record is often enough; at other times, more is needed. The following additional recommendations are based primarily on clinical experience and common sense.

Orchestrating Resources. If spiritual needs are identified, a decision must be made about whether the HP is capable of meeting those needs or whether referral is necessary. HPs will vary greatly in their interest, training, and experience in this area. Regardless, I believe that it is the *physician's* responsibility (as head of the health care team) to ensure that spiritual needs are met by someone, even though the physician will not likely be the person who actually meets those needs. A study of 160 primary care doctors revealed that 69 percent disagreed with the statement, "Only clergy should address religious issues."[7] Sometimes, relatively simple interventions by the physician or another HP are enough to resolve the issue. Listening with respect and concern may be all that is needed. Often, however, more extensive help is required, and few HPs have the time or training necessary to address spiritual needs in any depth (even those who are motivated to do so). For that reason, when complex spiritual issues are present, referral of the patient to pastoral care experts is necessary (after permission to do so has been obtained from the patient).

As emphasized throughout this book, professional chaplains are the true spiritual care experts in the health care setting (see chapter 7). A chaplain certified by the Association of Professional Chaplains (or by another recognized national chaplaincy organization) has gone through extensive training to meet the spiritual needs of medical or psychiatric patients. That training typically involves four years of college, three years of divinity school, and one or more years of clinical pastoral education in a hospital setting. Formal training is followed by written and oral board exams and a letter of recommendation by the chaplain's denominational office before certification is given. Since chaplains are the true specialists in this area, they should be fully utilized whenever possible. If chaplains are not available, then pastoral counselors or trained clergy from the patient's religious denomination should be consulted. Note, however, that many—perhaps most— community clergy have not received sufficient training to address the kinds of spiritual needs that arise in the medical setting. Thus, the chaplain or trained pastoral counselor may be the only person who can fully address the hospitalized patient's unique spiritual needs.

Some patients, however, may refuse to see the chaplain. As noted above, having a long-term relationship with an HP could make the patient feel more comfortable discussing religious worries or doubts with that person. Sometimes chaplains are not available at the critical time when spiritual issues arise, such as in the emergency room, in outpatient settings, or in chronic care settings such as rehabilitation centers or nursing homes. In such situations, the HP should take a few minutes to clarify concerns (by listening in a caring and supportive manner), and then later refer the patient to pastoral care experts for more definitive management. If the patient refuses to see the chaplain, and spiritual concerns are substantial, then repeated gentle and persuasive encouragement (without coercion) may help to change the patient's mind.

Other resources that patients may need are religious reading materials, access to religious services (hospital chapel or television), someone to contact their clergy, or time to pray with clergy or members of their religious group or family. These needs should be honored and the environment adapted so that they can be met. This is particularly true in the busy hospital setting, where routines often take precedent over patient need, especially in the area of spirituality. If this is not done, then patients may be prevented from gaining access to religious resources that they would ordinarily have if they were not sick and confined to an institutional setting (i.e., they will be forcibly *isolated* from spiritual resources). Institutions have an obligation to prevent such isolation, just as military and prison officials must provide soldiers or prisoners access to religious resources and freedom to practice their religion. Chapter 13 catalogues the many health-related practices that different religious traditions have, and these may be central to the well-being of the patient and family.

Support Spiritual Beliefs. As the HP takes the spiritual history and learns about how a patient's spiritual beliefs are used to cope with the medical illness, it is important to be respectful and seek understanding. Even if the patient's beliefs are unfamiliar to the HP, are different from what the HP believes, or even conflict with the medical, nursing, or rehabilitation care plan, the purpose is to *enter into the worldview of the patient* in order to understand why the patient believes as he or she does. (There is further discussion of this topic in chapter 6.)

If religious beliefs are not interfering with medical care, appear to be used by the patient to help with coping, and are not obviously pathological or harmful, then supporting religious beliefs and practices may be considered. This step is a bit more aggressive, and some HPs are uncomfortable with doing anything beyond taking a spiritual history, acknowledging and respecting the patient's beliefs, and, if necessary, making a referral. Others will feel more comfortable taking this next step. Because religious beliefs have been shown in numerous studies to facilitate patients' coping with medical illness, which may ultimately influence compliance with treatment and medical outcomes, I believe it is appropriate for the HP to support the religious beliefs of the patient that bring comfort, hope, and meaning. The goal of such support is not to make patients more religious or spiritual, but rather to reinforce an effective coping behavior that patients are using that may affect the outcome of the physical illness. The intention of the HP is always to maximize health, not promote religion. Chapter 1 summarizes evidence indicating that religious beliefs and practices often help patients cope better with illness, are associated with less depression, and may affect the course of the medical condition.

In order to enhance the religious patient's coping with illness, the HP may even point out that there is evidence from scientific research suggesting that religious beliefs help many patients to cope better and thereby can influence their health outcomes. Pointing this out to patients who are not religious, however, is inappropriate, and could be viewed as coercive. Remember that the HP is supporting beliefs and practices that are already being engaged in by the patient, not introducing new beliefs or encouraging practices that are foreign.

Keeping the support patient centered and ensuring that the goal of the support is health related are both crucial. The HP is nurturing and supporting the patient's own faith, whatever it is and however much of it there is—at all times being guided by cues from the patient. Inquiring about and addressing spiritual issues with patients is a bit like dancing. In ballroom dancing, one of the partners always leads. As the HP deals with spiritual issues, be sure that the patient is leading this dance and can stop the dance at any time.

Pray with Patients. The most controversial aspect of addressing spiritual issues in patient care is whether the HP should engage in spiritual activities with the patient, or whether this goes beyond the HP's responsibility and professional role. The most likely spiritual activity that HPs will be confronted with is praying with patients. There is no controversy if the HP prays silently for patients without their knowledge.[8] Any action beyond that, however, carries with it some risk—risk that some HPs believe is worth taking and others do not. On the one hand, when an HP prays with a religious patient, this can provide enormous comfort and support and strengthen the HP-patient relationship. On the other hand, HP-led prayer can also make the patient feel imposed upon, pressured, and uncomfortable. Some believe that this activity should never take place between a non-chaplain HP and patient,[9] and there are reports of patients' family members actually suing and winning cases against HPs when prayer is done inappropriately or indiscriminately (see chapter 5). Others believe that decisions on whether to pray with patients should be made on a case-by-case basis, since appropriateness greatly depends on the patient, the situation, and the HP (the next chapter includes a discussion about when praying with patients might be acceptable and when it is not). Who initiates such activity may be a key factor.

Patients are more likely to want to pray with HPs than vice versa. In fact, many HPs (especially physicians) are not aware that some patients might want this. A study of 160 randomly selected Illinois primary care physicians conducted in the mid-1980s revealed that only about one-third (37%) believed that patients might want to pray with them (this was in reference to patients who were older with severe or life-threatening medical illness).[10] When older patients in the same area were then asked if they would like their physicians to pray with them, 29 percent indicated "yes, somewhat," and 53 percent indicated "yes, very much." Only 5 percent of patients were definitely opposed.[11] As reviewed earlier, other studies in medical populations have likewise reported that between 28 percent and 67 percent of patients have positive attitudes toward prayer with physicians,[12] and 64 percent of the American populace believes that physicians should join patients in prayer if the patient asks.[13] This is especially true for patients with serious or terminal illnesses, when more than 50 percent of patients indicate that they would like their doctors to pray with them.[14]

Even in the mid-1980s, a significant proportion of primary care physicians reported having prayed with patients. In the study of Illinois physicians mentioned above,[15] one-third indicated that they had prayed with a patient at some time or another during their medical careers. Of those, only about 10 percent (6 physicians) reported that the prayer did not help the patient at all, whereas 34 percent indicated that it helped "somewhat," and 55 percent that it helped "a great deal." In a study of seventy-eight physicians in departments of internal medicine, neurology, surgery, and family medicine at a St. Louis academic medical center, 55 percent indicated that a patient had requested to pray with them in a non-crisis situation.[16] (If crisis situations had been included, the figure would have been considerably higher.) Thus, it appears that a significant proportion of patients would appreciate (and might ask their HPs) to pray with them, and that a significant proportion of HPs have prayed with patients, the majority reporting good results (based on studies of physicians).

Although I deal thoroughly in chapter 3 with the timing of and conditions necessary for HP-initiated and patient-initiated prayer, I will touch on a few aspects related to this now. There is concern that if an HP says a prayer with a patient out loud in public that there will be an "appearance of religious coercion" (even if the patient requests the prayer).[17] Ethicists with this belief insist that HP-led prayer is acceptable only if clergy are not readily available. Although I understand the concern, I do not agree with this viewpoint. In some circumstances, patients may not want to pray with unknown clergy, but prefer to pray with their HPs, whom they may have known for many years and have grown to trust. A patient may want to pray with the medical doctor or surgeon because he or she is in charge of the patient's care. Prayer with an HP may give the patient confidence that the HP is proceeding according to God's will and with God's blessing and guidance. Prayer does not have to be very complicated or sophisticated. Most HPs with little or no training are able to say a short, supportive, patient-centered prayer (see below). Another way to proceed if asked to pray by the patient is for the HP to encourage *the patient* to say the prayer, while the HP participates by being present. Some patients, however, will not be satisfied with this. Others may be so overwhelmed in crisis situations that they can't pray.

The vast majority of physicians agree that if the patient asks the physician to pray with him or her, then it is appropriate to do so.[18]

However, most patients don't know that prayer with their HPs is even possible. Because of the recent history of lack of HP involvement in religious activities with patients, many patients are scared to approach HPs about this. Therefore, I recommend that if HPs are willing to pray, they should inform patients about their willingness, but not initiate prayer at that time. If patients really want prayer, they will then be free to initiate a request during a future visit. This lets patients know that the HP is willing to pray with them, and gives them time to think about whether this is something they really want. If it is, then patients can bring up the subject themselves to the HP. This way, there is no coercion on the HP's part and the prayer request is always initiated by the patient.

How does an HP go about praying with a patient? Assuming that the conditions are met for the timing of prayer as outlined in chapter 3, the prayer should be short, supportive, and comforting. Its content should be consistent with the patient's religious beliefs and informed by what the patient wishes prayer for. The HP should always ask the patient what he or she would like prayer for. It is unwise and perhaps even rude for the HP to assume that he or she knows. Asking the patient about what the HP should pray about shows respect and humility. Furthermore, the HP will learn a lot from the patient's response to this question. What is the patient's first priority and greatest desire? It may not be for physical cure, but perhaps for the strength to cope or for the well-being of family members or friends. The HP should not assume anything in this regard.

Next, the HP might begin by taking the patient's hand, or by placing a hand on the patient's upper back or shoulder. This will depend on the comfort level of the HP and on the age and gender of the HP and patient. During the prayer, the HP may or may not decide to close his or her eyes. The prayer should probably last less than a minute. Long and complicated prayers said aloud by an HP with a patient in a health care setting are inappropriate. If the patient believes in a personal God, then it is appropriate to emphasize God's love for that person, asking for peace, comfort, and strength for the patient and the family to help them endure through the illness, and wisdom and skill for the doctor to treat the patient's medical or surgical condition effectively.

There is some controversy about whether or not to pray for physical healing (given the disappointment that may result if physical cure does not result), and it is always best to discuss this beforehand when asking what the patient wishes prayer for. Many patients appreciate prayer for physical healing, so this should not be ignored. Some HPs may even pray that the medications they prescribe will have a more powerful effect, helping the body or mind to heal rapidly and completely.

Prescribe Religious Activities. If the effects of religious beliefs and practices on health are equivalent to not smoking cigarettes or to physical exercise, perhaps HPs should prescribe religious activities?[19] Should doctors urge nonreligious patients to become religious, pray, attend religious services more regularly, or begin a study of religious scriptures to maintain or improve their health? In almost every case, this goes beyond what HPs should do and has serious potential for coercion and infringement on patient rights. First of all, religion is a sensitive and deeply personal area of patients' lives, and HPs cannot ethically pressure patients how to believe or behave in this area. Furthermore, there is no evidence from clinical trials that if patients become more religious *only in order to be healthier* that better health will result. The research shows that persons who are religious may have better health outcomes. These persons are usually religious for religious reasons (not health reasons). Better health is an unintended consequence of devout religious belief and practice. Finally, prescriptions for greater religious activity for health reasons would involve an "extrinsic" use of religion to acquire a nonspiritual end, and extrinsic religiosity is not usually associated with better health (and often quite the opposite). Nevertheless, there will always be gray areas that need to be handled on a case-by-case basis (see chapter 5).

Linking with Religious Communities. While not all HPs will decide to pray with patients, there are other spiritual interventions that can help improve the health of patients and the quality of care they receive. As noted in chapter 1, as health care begins to shift more and more away from costly institutional settings, HPs and health care systems need to consider linking with religious groups through "parish nurses" (or lay leaders) to more fully address the health needs of patients and families in the community. Although this applies to all Americans (70% of whom belong to a church, synagogue, or temple), such linkages are particularly important for meeting health-education and disease-prevention goals in minority communities, whose populations are often very religious and yet experience high rates of disease and poor disease outcomes. Negative health practices (smoking, alcohol, and drug use), low rates of disease screening (breast, cervical, prostate, and colon cancer; hypertension and diabetes), lack of information about diet, exercise, and weight control, and poor access to health care are largely responsible for the health disparities in these communities. Programs developed within religious communities to address such health issues have been effective in many cases.[20]

HPs are now experiencing more and more difficulty getting patients into the hospital unless they are severely ill, often having to send sick patients home from the office because there is no other place to send them. These trends will increase over the next thirty to forty years as the over sixty-five population in the United States increases from the current 35 million to greater than 75 million, as baby boomers reach their retirement years starting in 2011.[21] According to an article written in the highly respected journal *Science,* Ed Schneider (dean of the Andrus Gerontology Center at University of Southern California) indicates that if we simply continue on our current trajectory, then many baby boomers will be spending their later years in city parks and on city streets because there will be nowhere to provide care for them.[22]

Religious communities have always been the first to meet the needs of the poor, destitute, and downcast members of society, and historically were the first to meet the health care needs of persons in the community who couldn't afford medical care. Religious communities could be a source of healthy volunteers to provide practical services for sick members and respite for their families. Working with parish nurses (registered nurses who are members of a religious community and provide health leadership there) can help ensure that the medical plan for a patient is carried out, that worsening illness is identified early, and that appropriate follow-up is obtained. Parish nurses can also mobilize and train volunteers, as well as initiate health education and health screening programs to maintain wellness.[23]

Working with religious communities to help meet the health care needs of patients after they are discharged back into the community, then, seems beneficial to all. In addition to maintaining open lines of communication with religious communities, physicians and other HPs can act as consultants to congregational health programs or participate in them by providing lectures and teaching health classes.

SUMMARY AND CONCLUSIONS

Addressing the spiritual needs of patients means that HPs must learn to take a spiritual history in a manner that is patient centered and respects the patient's beliefs. A spiritual history provides information relevant to the care of the patient and communicates to the patient that the HP is open to communicating about needs in this area. For all but the most simple of spiritual needs that arise during such spiritual screenings, referral to professional chaplains and pastoral counselors should be the rule. HPs may consider supporting the religious beliefs and activities that patients find helpful and are not obviously harmful. In special circumstances, the HP may consider praying with a patient, although this activity is more risky than either assessing spiritual needs or supporting the patient's beliefs. Finally, lines of communication should be kept open between HPs and religious communities in order to mobilize resources to meet the patient's health care needs after discharge from the hospital or clinic. Working with parish nurses and even volunteering time to support congregational health programs are other ways that HPs can meet the physical, psychological, and spiritual needs of patients, both within and outside health care settings.

CHAPTER 3

WHEN TO INCLUDE SPIRITUALITY

The *timing* of spiritual assessment and support is essential. When is the best time to take a spiritual history? At what point during the medical assessment should this be done, and why? How often should spiritual histories be repeated? When should an HP support the religious beliefs of patients? Do certain kinds of patients and situations call for spiritual assessment and support, whereas others do not? When and under what circumstances is it appropriate to pray with patients? Little systematic research exists on which to base recommendations, although clinical experience and common sense will once again be our guide.

IMPORTANCE OF TIMING

A patient is in the intensive care unit, coming out of anesthesia following a major life-threatening surgical operation. Another patient is in the coronary care unit recovering from a myocardial infarction. A third patient is in the emergency room immediately following a car accident in which serious injuries have occurred. Raising spiritual issues at these times will probably elicit the same response from each patient above—*fear.* Remember that in the old days (and in more recent times as well, in some cultures), when a priest or minister was brought in to see a sick patient, it was to give last rites because death was near.[1] Bringing up spiritual issues at these times, then, may send the wrong message to the patient—that his or her condition is hopeless and that nothing more can be done. Of course, if death is imminent or spiritual issues come up in such situations, the HP must be ready to address them. Even in such cases, however, there is no need to arouse unnecessary fear. A brief introduction (as described in chapter 2) explaining why these questions are being asked will usually allay anxiety. Sometimes, though, it is better to wait until things are more stable before taking a spiritual history, particularly if there is no urgency to do so.

A healthy patient comes to the doctor's office for the removal of a wart or mole. A man with a cold comes to see an HP requesting medicine to relieve unpleasant physical symptoms. A young man comes in for a physical exam for health insurance purposes. These are not times when it is necessary to bring up spiritual issues. Each of these patients has a specific agenda for the visit. Such patients do not expect questions about their spirituality and may not appreciate the HP raising spiritual issues at this time. Doing so, in fact, may confuse and upset them.

A nurse is taking the history from a patient being seen in the emergency room to sew up a laceration obtained by punching his hand through glass. A physician is covering for one of her partners who is away on vacation, and is seeing the partner's patient for a follow-up exam after hospital discharge. A neurologist sees a patient for Parkinson's disease who is referred by the patient's primary care physician. In most of these situations, the HP and the patient have never seen each other before and will probably never see each other again. There is no stable relationship (past or future) between patient and the HP, and no real reason for the HP to be aware of the patient's spiritual beliefs.

Timing of the spiritual history and other spiritual interventions is crucial.

WHEN TO DO A SPIRITUAL HISTORY

There are specific times when a spiritual history is indicated and can be done in such a way that it does not surprise patients, take them off guard, or send unintended messages, and when there is sufficient time to address both medical and spiritual concerns. The best times to do an initial spiritual history are (1) when taking the medical history during a new patient evaluation; (2) when taking the medical history while admitting a patient to the hospital, nursing home, hospice, or palliative care setting; and (3) when doing a health maintenance visit as part of a well-person evaluation. In each of these instances, the HP will have more time than during a rushed ten-minute office visit.

New Patient Evaluation. When a new patient comes for an initial visit to a primary care physician, a complete history and physical exam are usually done in the office. Part of the medical history is the social history. The social history usually comes after the past medical history and before the physical exam. It typically consists of asking questions about the patient's job, education, members of the family, and other support systems. A brief spiritual history fits very nicely at the end of the social history in the section exploring other support systems. Questions about religious denomination, whether the patient is a member of a faith community, whether religious beliefs provide comfort, and how such beliefs might affect medical decisions—all flow quite naturally after inquiring about family and friends. As noted in the last chapter, information learned from the spiritual history should be recorded in the medical record so that it can be referred to when necessary. Doing a spiritual history at this time, particularly if preceded by a brief introduction, will not alarm the patient as it might if spiritual issues were raised during more acute medical or surgical situations.

Admission to the Hospital. Patients with serious illness requiring acute hospitalization or nursing home admission should also have a spiritual assessment completed during the admitting history, particularly if this has not been done within the past six months. Often, however, the admitting HP is not the patient's primary care provider. Many hospitals now hire specialized physicians called hospitalists to provide the medical care for all hospitalized patients. Since these HPs and hospital nurses usually don't have access to the primary care physician's records that contain this information, the spiritual history should be completed on admission, since that information may affect decisions made in the hospital. In case of a surgical admission, the same is true for the HP who does the admitting history and will be the main person taking care of the patient or making the medical decisions. If the patient is being admitted for a diagnostic or therapeutic procedure that requires only an overnight stay, a spiritual history is less urgent, although this depends on the kind of procedure being done and for what reason. A spiritual history should also be considered for all patients newly admitted to a nursing home, to home health care, or to a hospice program. Again, this is best done as part of the social history.

Health Maintenance Visit. Many people have yearly physical examinations that focus on disease prevention and health maintenance. More time is usually set aside for a health maintenance visit than for a visit dealing with an acute problem. The HP may ask about different health habits and inquire about the patient's family, job, and life stressors. A spiritual history taken at this time fits nicely after questions about family, job, and sources of stress. Again, raising spiritual issues at this time is less likely to alarm the patient than if brought up when the patient is deathly ill. Regardless of when the spiritual history is taken, medical issues should always be competently and completely addressed before turning to spiritual issues.

REPEATING THE SPIRITUAL HISTORY

Care needs to be taken, particularly in acute hospital settings, so that different HPs do not repeat the spiritual history during the same admission. For example, what would happen if the primary care physician, hospitalist, surgeon, nurse, and social worker all felt obligated to take a spiritual history? This would likely disturb the patient with repetitive questions. Thus, a good general rule is that whoever is taking primary responsibility for the patient in the hospital should be the person who takes the spiritual history and records it in the medical record. This is the physician. Such notes need not be lengthy, but simply indicate that a spiritual history has been taken, whether or not spiritual matters are important to the patient, and how religious beliefs may influence medical decisions or conflict with the medical plan. Nurses, who often do their own spiritual histories, should be aware if the physician has already completed one and proceed tactfully (and vice versa). As indicated in the last chapter, having a special section in the medical record for this purpose improves communication and avoids repetition.

How often should a spiritual history be repeated by the same HP? After a spiritual history has been taken and documented in the patient's outpatient or inpatient medical record, several months or years may pass before the spiritual history needs to be reviewed or updated, depending on the patient's health condition. The primary indication for an update is when there is a major change in the patient's health, social, or living environment (e.g., onset of a serious illness, serious accident, loss of a spouse or child, relocation to nursing home, and so forth). Admission to the hospital is a good reason to review the spiritual history. In general, common sense and need for information should always dictate the frequency of spiritual assessments.

SUPPORTING RELIGIOUS ACTIVITIES

Besides taking a spiritual history, the HP may decide to support the religious beliefs or activities of the patient to improve the patient's ability to cope with illness and changes the illness has caused. Timing here is also important. This is best done while taking the spiritual history, when the patient is talking about the role that religion plays in his or her coping. Paying undivided attention to the patient's answers and providing positive verbal and nonverbal responses are ways to show support and respect. If the HP learns that spiritual factors are important for coping, then this information may be utilized at other times in the future when helping the patient adjust to a particular situation.

If the patient expresses current or past interest in religious beliefs and activities but regrets that such activities are no longer engaged in or cannot be engaged in due to health or transportation problems, then the HP may gently explore with the patient whether he or she would like to increase involvement in this area and how barriers to this activity might be overcome. When supporting spiritual involvement, however, it is a fine line to walk to avoid inducing guilt or making the patient feel uncomfortable over lack of involvement. The HP must at all times guard against the latter and back off whenever the patient indicates that he or she does not wish to engage in such activities or seems uncomfortable with the discussion.

If the patient expresses no interest in religious or spiritual matters, then there is no room to support or encourage these activities. As noted earlier, the HP may decide to inquire about social or altruistic activities more generally, without referring to religion or spirituality. Another alternative for the nonreligious patient might be mind-body meditation techniques to elicit the "relaxation response," which has been shown to lower blood pressure, reduce anxiety, and positively affect neuroendocrine and immune functioning.[2]

REFERRING TO CLERGY

If spiritual needs are identified that are not readily addressed by the HP through listening and support, then a chaplain or pastoral referral is necessary. This is particularly true if the patient comes from a different religious background and culture than the HP. Referral should probably come sooner than later. While this depends on the HP's comfort, training, and expertise in this area, the HP will seldom have the kind of training a chaplain has. Many HPs will feel unprepared, uncomfortable, and lack the time or interest to address the spiritual needs of patients, and should not feel guilty about referring these patients (after taking a spiritual history) to the true experts in these matters. The HP should also attempt to get to know the chaplain staff, which will help the

HP learn about their strengths and weaknesses and also acquire information about other pastoral resources in the area.

PRAYING WITH PATIENTS

When is praying with patients acceptable? This depends on whether the prayer is HP initiated or patient initiated. As I indicated in the last chapter, some experts advise that HPs never initiate spiritual activities with patients, and instead rely on the patient to take the first step. Because of the difference in power status between patient and HP, there is a risk that coercion may enter the picture whenever the HP initiates such activities. This is because it is difficult for the patient to refuse such a request, particularly in the hospital, where patients may not be able to pick their HPs. This concern is particularly important since surveys indicate that many patients don't wish to pray with their HPs. There may be times, however, when the HP will want to initiate the prayer, particularly when the HP senses that a religious patient is undergoing a great deal of distress.

HP-Initiated Prayer

If HPs decide to initiate prayer with patients, they should proceed with caution and only when certain conditions are met:

1. A thorough spiritual history has been taken so that the HP is certain that the patient will appreciate and welcome such an action.

2. The HP has the same religious background as the patient (e.g., Christian, Jewish, Buddhist, Muslim, Hindu).

3. There is a spiritual need present and the situation calls for prayer.

Spiritual History Has Been Taken. After taking a complete spiritual history, the HP knows beyond doubt that the patient would appreciate an offer to pray. "Beyond doubt." In other words, the patient is as certain to say "yes" (and to truly appreciate it) as a teenage basketball player would say "yes" to an offer to shoot hoops with Michael Jordan, as certain as a scientist would agree to accept the Nobel prize, as certain as a Virginia resident would take the winning ticket for the state lottery. The point is clear. The HP needs to know the answer to the question before the question is asked. If the patient is heavily depending on religious belief to cope and the HP supports that belief by offering to pray, then this will help reinforce the patient's ability to cope and provide comfort. If the patient is not using religion to cope, then this increases the risk that the HP's offer to pray will be perceived as intrusive and possibly upsetting. Unless a thorough spiritual history is taken, the HP cannot know how the patient will react.

Same Religious Background. If the HP is from a different religious tradition than the patient, the risk of coercion and undue influence increases (whether intended or not). The content of the prayer is usually influenced by the religious tradition from which it emerges. For example, praying to God presupposes the existence of a personal God who listens and responds to prayer. While Christians, Jews, and Muslims may have no problem with this, a Buddhist patient might. Furthermore, among Christians there are disagreements about whether one should pray for divine intervention for physical healing or pray for "God's will" in a situation. Thus, even when religious background is similar, doctrinal differences may influence the content of the prayer. Lack of similar religious background, however, is a relative contraindication to prayer, not an absolute one,[3] and this applies only to HP-initiated prayer. There may be rare instances where a Jewish or Muslim HP may initiate a prayer with a Christian patient, if other conditions are present, but considerable risk of coercion remains, and this must be carefully guarded against.

Spiritual Need Is Present. Unless HPs advertise it as part of their practices and patients are made aware of this policy before being seen, they should not initiate prayer with patients as a matter of routine. Prayer should be reserved for crises or circumstances where neither the patient nor the HP is in control of the outcome—and the outcome is a serious one (when illness threatens life or way of life of the patient or his or her loved ones). Initiating prayer with patients, if done at all, should not be done lightly, and the decision should be made on a case-by-case basis. The circumstances should be of a nature that it is obvious that the patient is dealing with a major life crisis with spiritual implications. As indicated above for the spiritual history, prayer should not be initiated when a patient comes in for a flu shot, treatment of a minor infection, or sprained ankle. In the end, however, the patient should determine whether a spiritual need is present that prayer would be helpful in addressing.

Even if all three conditions above are met, the HP should continue to remain sensitive and draw cues from the patient throughout the prayer activity. The HP should ensure that the patient feels in control at all times. If HPs want to be cautious and avoid having to initiate prayer, as pointed out earlier, they may simply inform religious patients that they are open to praying with patients and encourage them to make a request at some later time if this is something that patients desire. If these simple basic rules are followed, HP-initiated prayer will almost always be deeply appreciated by patients.

The specialty of the HP may also make a difference in how appropriate it is to initiate a spiritual activity like prayer with

patients. A primary care physician who is treating a psychologically healthy and stable patient who is coping with a difficult
medical problem may suggest a prayer with less risk than might
a psychiatrist who is treating a psychologically frail patient with
borderline personality disorder. Although all HPs need to worry
about this to some extent, the psychiatrist, mental health counselor, or psychiatric nurse must be more cautious about broach-
ing boundaries in relationships with patients than do the primary
care physician, the surgeon, or the medical nurse. More will be
said about boundary issues in chapters 5 and 11.

Patient-initiated Prayer

This is less controversial than HP-initiated prayer, although as
pointed out in the last chapter, medical ethicists have concerns
about HP-led prayer even when the patient takes the first step.[4]
There is certainly less risk of coercion if the patient makes the first
move. In some circumstances, it may be most appropriate to have
the patient say the prayer. This is perhaps best when the HP feels
uneasy about praying with patients or is not entirely familiar with
the patient's religious beliefs. In those cases, as the patient prays,
the HP should sit nearby perhaps joining hands with the patient,
and conclude the prayer by saying "Amen" (what is appropriate
here may vary by religious tradition). Patient-led prayer, however, may not have the same impact as HP-led prayer, and many
religious patients prefer the latter. The HP can always ask the
patient for his or her preference, although the HP will then have
to be prepared to say the prayer if that is what the patient wants.

What about an HP who is an agnostic or an atheist? Is it necessary to comply with the patient's request even when the HP
doesn't believe in prayer? Is it not dishonest to conceal from the
patient the HP's lack of belief? Again, opinions by experts vary,[5]

but it seems to me that if an HP can bring comfort to a patient by saying "Amen" at the end of a patient-led prayer, then I can't think of a good reason not to do so—regardless of the HP's personal beliefs. Saying "Amen" does not acknowledge belief in God, Muhammad, Buddha, or anything supernatural. It simply means "let it be so." Let it be so that the patient's request for health and healing is granted (through medicine, religion, or the random forces of nature).

Our role as HPs is to cure sometimes, relieve often, *comfort always*. If a little child who is sick and afraid asks her doctor to examine her teddy bear to be sure he's okay, would the doctor refuse? No, because he wants to comfort the little girl. Showing kindness and concern for the things that are important to our patients is really what matters here.

SUMMARY AND CONCLUSIONS

This chapter examined the timing of spiritual interventions. HPs should not conduct a spiritual history on an outpatient coming in for a wart removal, a cold, a routine Pap smear, or other minor problem, nor should they conduct such assessments in intensive care or emergency room settings—unless the situation clearly indicates that spiritual needs are present. The best times for conducting a spiritual history are during a new patient evaluation, particularly for patients with severe or chronic illness that may challenge their coping abilities; when patients are admitted to the hospital for a new problem or exacerbation of an old one, to a nursing home or other chronic institutional setting, or to hospice or a palliative care setting; during a health maintenance visit of a healthy patient; or whenever medical decisions need to be made that may be influenced by religious beliefs. Taking a spiritual history is most important when a serious acute or chronic medical illness is threatening life or quality of life, when a major psychosocial stressor is present that involves loss or change (e.g., divorce, bereavement, sick family member, and so forth), or when the patient is about to undergo a major surgical operation or other procedure where the outcome is uncertain and the patient is having difficulty coping. Having knowledge about the spiritual resources of the patient prior to the onset or sudden worsening of a medical condition is always preferable to having to initiate a spiritual history at the time of the acute event.

Spiritual support may be provided during a spiritual history and at other times as the situation warrants. Unless obviously harmful, HPs should feel free to provide simple support for religious beliefs and activities that the patient finds helpful in coping with illness, although they should always be ready to refer patients to clergy with experience meeting spiritual needs. On some occasions and under certain carefully defined circumstances, an HP may decide to pray with a patient, either initiating the prayer him- or herself or agreeing to pray at the patient's request. To minimize risk of coercion, it is safest when the patient initiates the request for prayer. However, before some religious patients will ask, the HP may need to indicate that he or she is open to praying with patients. Time spent addressing spiritual issues, however, should never replace the time necessary to comprehensively address patients' medical needs.

CHAPTER 4

WHAT MIGHT RESULT?

In practical terms, what might result from HPs' addressing the spiritual needs of patients—taking a spiritual
history, supporting religious beliefs, and mobilizing spiritual support by others? What difference could this make
in the quality of care that patients receive and in the
medical outcomes that result? While there has been only
one systematic study examining what happens when HPs
(physicians, in that study) address spiritual issues, there
is information from that study and related research to
hypothesize the kinds of health effects that might occur.
Addressing spiritual issues could make a difference (either
positive or negative) in a range of outcomes relevant to
the health and care of the patient.

Conducting a spiritual history and ensuring that spiritual needs are met may affect the patient's ability to cope
and quality of life, the HP-patient relationship, patient
compliance, and the overall course of illness and response
to treatment. Communicating with, referring to, and inter-

acting with clergy in hospital and community settings may further influence health outcomes by affecting the quality of support and monitoring that patients receive in their communities. And the patient may not be the only one who benefits. The HP may experience the satisfaction of treating the whole person, find his or her work more meaningful, and see patients who are happier with their care. The results, however, might not always be positive—and that too must be considered.

ABILITY TO COPE

The impact of belief should not be underestimated. Whether it's religious belief, belief in the doctor, belief in the medical treatment, or any strongly held conviction, belief influences motivations and emotions in powerful ways. This idea underlies the rationale for one of the most common forms of psychotherapy used to treat depression and anxiety in the United States today: cognitive therapy. According to cognitive theory, dysfunctional beliefs and pessimistic thoughts lie at the root of negative emotions such as depression and anxiety. Cognitive therapy seeks to alter dysfunctional beliefs and maladaptive cognitions so that a patient's interpretations and views of the world become both more realistic and positive. The rule according to the theory is that positive emotions follow positive beliefs. Religious beliefs are usually rooted in a positive, optimistic worldview.[1] For example, most members of monotheistic religious traditions believe that a benevolent creator rules the universe and responds to human prayer, that all things (even negative events and difficult life situations) have meaning and purpose, and that after death there is hope of eternal life, happiness, and the end of suffering. Such beliefs enable people to integrate and adapt to negative life circumstances more easily, and motivate others in their family and community to help them. In particular, religious beliefs give sick patients hope that may help them to persevere in difficult circumstances that are not changing.

If the patient is relying on religious beliefs and practices to cope, then any action by an HP that acknowledges and strengthens those beliefs will likely bolster the patient's ability to cope. Studies tell us that religious beliefs and practices are indeed associated with better coping, less depression, and greater well-being in those with significant health problems (chapter 1). Deep intrinsic religious motivation predicts faster recovery from depression in patients with medical illness. Religious interventions that utilize and support the beliefs of the patient result in more speedy resolution of depression and anxiety.[2] Again, affirming the religious beliefs of patients will help them to more effectively use those beliefs in adapting to life changes caused by health problems. On the other hand, if religious beliefs or conflicts are causing stress rather than providing support, then finding someone who can help the patient work through these issues becomes urgent.

How might taking a brief, screening spiritual history influence the coping process? First, when an HP asks about religious beliefs, religious patients have an opportunity to recount or witness to the HP how faith has helped them to cope. The use of religion as a coping behavior is reinforced by the act of verbalizing the benefits; it makes the person more aware and conscious of those benefits. Second, most patients feel that if an HP asks about something, then it must be important—since HPs don't have much time and they ask only about important things. The fact that religious beliefs and activities are important enough for the HP to ask about sends a powerful message that further reinforces their effectiveness (and if those beliefs are causing distress, validates the need to ask for help in this area). If the HP also supports beliefs and practices that provide comfort, then this gives those beliefs the "authority" of medical approval, strengthening them even further. As the belief gains power, it has more and more potency to affect adjustment and coping. Of course, there is always the possibility that a non-religious patient will feel uncomfortable by such questions, and for that reason, great care must be taken to quickly and smoothly switch to another topic if religion or spirituality isn't that patient's cup of tea. This very valid concern, however, is not sufficient to deprive the vast majority of patients who are religious or spiritual of the comfort that inquiring about and supporting their beliefs could bring.

Only one study to date has examined the effects of inquiring about spiritual issues on patient outcomes. As briefly described earlier, the Oncologist Assisted Spiritual Intervention Study (OASIS) involved 118 consecutive outpatients with cancer seen in the offices of four oncologists (2 Christians, 1 Hindu, and 1 Sikh).[3] Patients were alternatively assigned to either the intervention group or a control group in order to minimize burden on any one oncologist. The FACT-G (quality of life), Brief Symptom Inventory-Depression, and Primary Care Assessment Survey Interpersonal and Communication Scales were administered before and three weeks after the intervention. The OASIS intervention (which involved a bit more than a spiritual history) took on average six minutes to administer, and increased the length of the visit by 1.7 minutes (from 13.1 to 14.8 minutes) (these were outpatients). In 85 percent of cases, oncologists felt comfortable administering the OASIS interview, and in 76 percent of cases, the patient indicated that it was useful. At the three-week follow-up, compared to the control group, the intervention group had a significant reduction in depressive symptoms ($p < 0.01$), improved sense of interpersonal caring from the physician ($p < 0.05$), and increased functional well-being

($p < 0.001$). Authors concluded that the OASIS interview had a positive impact on the perception of care and well-being of patients.

In 1910, legendary physician William Osler (then at Oxford University) wrote a short article in the *British Medical Journal* entitled "The Faith That Heals."[4] In the first sentence, Osler writes, "Nothing in life is more wonderful than faith—the one great moving force which we can neither weigh in the balance nor test in the crucible." Indeed, whatever we as HPs can do to support the faith of our patients, it is in their best interests that we do so.

HEALTH PROFESSIONAL–PATIENT RELATIONSHIP

The most important component of the HP-patient relationship is trust. The HP's recognition and support of a patient's religious belief, as noted above, helps strengthen that belief. It also does something else, however. Seeing that the HP recognizes and values what for many is central to their hope and sense of meaning enables the patient to place greater trust in the HP. This is primarily true for religious patients whose beliefs are important to them and their ability to cope. For many patients (more than 40% in some hospital settings; see chapter 1), there is nothing more important in helping them cope than their religious beliefs. These patients put great value and trust in their beliefs because those beliefs have helped them get through difficult situations in the past. If an HP validates the beliefs, this not only empowers the patient but also enables the patient to more fully place his or her trust in the HP and in the treatment plan. The bond between patient and HP becomes stronger, reinforced by a common belief system about what is important to healing.

We know that if a patient believes in the HP and believes in the treatment, the treatment will be more effective. The placebo response is based on the belief of the patient in the treatment. Combine the placebo effect with the actual therapeutic effect, and the effectiveness of treatment is magnified. Although the placebo response has its greatest effect on psychological or emotional states (indeed, it is not uncommon in antidepressant treatment studies to have placebo response rates of more than 40%), placebos also affect the way that physical illnesses respond to treatment. Thus, the patient's belief in the treatment may cause actual physiological changes that move the patient toward recovery.

By asking about the patient's religious beliefs in a respectful manner, the HP indicates a desire to understand an important part of who that person is. If the HP then supports those beliefs, the patient's trust in the HP may be amplified. If the HP agrees to pray with the religious patient when requested, that further confirms that the HP can be trusted. If so, the HP can utilize not only the power of medical therapies to affect health outcomes but also the power of the patient's belief and trust. Again, this applies mostly to religious patients.

COMPLIANCE

We know that compliance is strongly related to a patient's trust in the HP. In a study of 7,204 adults employed by the Commonwealth of Massachusetts, the physician's whole-person knowledge of the patient and the patient's trust in the physician were the variables most strongly associated with adherence to treatment.[5] With other factors equal, adherence rates were 2.6 times higher among patients whose physicians had whole-person knowledge scores in the ninety-fifth percentile compared with the fifth percentile (44.0% adherence vs. 16.8% adherence, $p < 0.001$).

Taking a spiritual history and addressing the patient's spiritual concerns can have a positive impact on compliance. First, address-ing spiritual issues makes patients (especially religious patients) feel like the HP is addressing them as whole persons. Consequently, the patient is more satisfied and the HP develops increased cred-ibility in the patient's eyes. Greater trust increases the likelihood that the patient will follow the HP's recommendations,[6] such as taking medication as prescribed, making behavioral changes, and complying with other aspects of the treatment plan. In addition to the randomized clinical trial (OASIS study) described above that documented improvement in the doctor-patient relationship after a spiritual history, other research indicates that religious persons in general tend to be more compliant with prescribed medication and with keeping doctor visits.[7] Patients who are treated as whole persons, that is, who have their spiritual needs addressed, will feel more obligated to continue treatment, even when it takes a lot of effort to comply and the benefits are not yet evident.

Second, if patients feel that the HP understands their religious beliefs or struggles and is receptive to discussing those beliefs, they will be more likely to tell the HP about religious beliefs that conflict with prescribed treatments or use of religious therapies instead of medical treatment. For example, a patient attends a healing service at church and decides to stop all medication because she now believes she is healed. If the HP makes an effort to enter into the spiritual worldview of the patient, the patient will be more likely to trust the HP in this area and share experi-ences. Having such information will enable the HP to follow the patient more carefully, with full knowledge of what is going on.

MOBILIZING COMMUNITY SUPPORT

Communicating with and referring to clergy in hospital and community settings can influence health care by affecting the quality of support that patients receive after leaving the clinician's office or discharge from the hospital, as well as improve timely referrals for necessary medical care.

First, if HPs become acquainted with community clergy when clergy are visiting patients in the hospital, they will find that clergy are more likely to support them and the treatments they prescribe. Clergy are also ideally positioned to reinforce the need for regular medical attention. If patients are aware that their clergy know and trust their HPs, then this will help patients to do likewise.

Second, the HP (with consent from the patient) may alert the patient's clergy about the patient's health care needs after an office visit or hospital discharge. This will enable the clergy to mobilize resources in the religious community to provide necessary emotional and spiritual support as well as practical services (e.g., respite services, meals, transportation) for the patient and family.

Third, clergy will be more likely to refer members of their congregation to the HP for health care, improving the promptness of attention to medical problems. HPs who have relationships with community clergy can also influence disease screening and healthy lifestyle practices of church members by encouraging health ministries programs at the congregation level and participating in them.

For example, at Methodist Health System in Dallas, Texas, there is a regular monthly meeting of forty to fifty physicians and forty to fifty clergy. They usually eat together, listen to a speaker, and then talk about various health issues that are of mutual concern. This has resulted in physicians and clergy understanding better what the other profession has to offer and how they can assist one another, and has helped to develop relationships that facilitate referrals and communications, making a true integration of spirituality into health care possible.

COURSE OF ILLNESS

Addressing spiritual issues may affect the overall course of medical or surgical illness and response to treatment (see chapter 1). This is accomplished by each of the potential benefits described above: improving the patient's ability to cope, enhancing the HP-patient relationship, and mobilizing support and disease monitoring at the community level.

First, because of the powerful influence that beliefs have in relieving stress, decreasing depression, and increasing hope, addressing spiritual issues may help to activate or maintain the body's natural systems of healing (neuroendocrine, immune, and circulatory systems). Sick patients who are experiencing a great deal of stress, anxiety, or depression have been shown to have longer hospital stays and greater mortality.[8] Psychosocial stress has even been found to slow down the speed of wound healing. It does so by altering the immune-mediated cascade of physiological events necessary for wound closure to take place.[9] Thus, psychosocial stress can prolong recovery after accidents or surgery and perhaps even increase the risk of infection. Anything that improves the patient's ability to cope with illness will reduce anxiety and increase hope, thus likely improving physical health outcomes as well. By supporting religious beliefs that help patients cope with illness and by helping patients work through stressful spiritual problems (usually by referral to professional chaplains), the HP may be performing important interventions with lasting medical consequences.

Second, treating the whole person by addressing spiritual aspects of illness increases the patient's satisfaction with treatment and trust in the HP. Level of trust, as pointed out earlier, strongly predicts compliance with treatment. Better adherence to the medical regimen, in turn, will improve disease outcomes.

Third, having greater confidence in the HP, the patient will have greater belief in the efficacy of treatment that the HP prescribes, magnifying the placebo effect, as discussed earlier. Research has shown that when a patient believes in the treatment, this increases the likelihood that the treatment will be effective (whether the treatment is actually effective or not).[10]

Fourth, by increasing the support that patients receive from their religious communities in terms of spiritual, psychological, social, and practical day-to-day help, this will further improve coping with illness by both patient and family. It will also help to ensure that medical therapies are complied with and prompt medical attention is sought when necessary. Thus, by addressing patients' spiritual issues and beginning a dialogue with community clergy, the HP can both directly and indirectly affect the course of illness.

BENEFITS TO THE HEALTH PROFESSIONAL

Although the reason for including spirituality in patient care is for the patient's well-being, HPs themselves may also unintentionally benefit from addressing the spiritual needs of patients. Because of the demands of both the outpatient clinic and the acute hospital setting, there is a temptation for busy HPs to run patients through like cattle—focusing only on their biological needs. As health care systems have become more and more concerned with the bottom line, HPs have become more pressured to increase their efficiency at seeing patients. That increased efficiency, however, has come at a cost—a cost not only to patients but to HPs as well.

The fact is that most of us don't become HPs for the money. If highly intelligent, talented young people worked twelve to sixteen hours a day, seven days a week, for seven to ten years to become business professionals, they would earn a lot more money than if they spent that time training to become a health professional. No, most of us become HPs because we want to help people, because we want to make a difference in people's lives and in the world around us. Sometimes, though, the training of HPs and the rigors of daily care for patients stamp out that idealism. When this happens, HPs begin to experience emptiness and lack of fulfillment in what they are doing, which may lead them to question their choice of profession.

HPs who begin to address the spiritual needs of patients sometimes experience an arousal of that buried sense of idealism that drove them to become HPs in the first place. No longer are they simply technicians caring for or fixing a physical body like a mechanic fixes a broken-down car. Rather, they become healers in the true sense of the word. As HPs begin to treat their patients as whole persons, they find themselves also becoming more complete and satisfied in their professional lives.

NEGATIVE CONSEQUENCES

This discussion so far has described only the positive consequences of addressing religious or spiritual issues in patient care. Could there also be negative results? The OASIS study described earlier reported that in 15 percent of cases, the physician did not feel comfortable administering the spiritual history, and in 24 percent of cases, the patient didn't find the spiritual history useful (bear in mind that two of the four physicians applying the intervention were non-Christian and the vast majority of patients were Christian, which could have inflated these figures).[11] Other than this study, no other systematic research exists that documents negative consequences. However, there are some sobering anecdotes that I have heard about that underscore the need for HPs to proceed intelligently, gently, and cautiously in this area. (The next two chapters further address issues of professional boundaries and religious harm.)

The first case involves a psychiatrist who prayed with a patient as part of his work in the Texas state mental health system. It is unclear whether the psychiatrist initiated the prayer, the patient requested it, or the psychiatrist took a spiritual history beforehand or obtained consent from the patient (probably not). In any event, the prayer apparently confused the patient, who told his family about it. When the family sued, the jury ruled against the psychiatrist and in favor of the family. Sadly, this case caused so much fear locally that it led to a number of psychiatric departments advising staff and residents not to address spiritual issues with patients.

A second case involves a woman whose physician made a diagnosis of metastatic lung cancer. She was very distraught. Her son had also recently been diagnosed with AIDS. Sensing how upset she was, her physician asked if he could say a prayer for her. She said, "Absolutely not," and got up and abruptly left the office. The physician never saw her again. A spiritual history might have helped in this situation by revealing the patient's experiences with and feelings about religion. That may have alerted the physician not to proceed with his offer to pray (although the patient may have also been upset by the spiritual history). There is a natural tendency for patients to ask "Why me?" when they are in the midst of agonizing circumstances. They may feel angry with

God for allowing them to suffer so deeply or for not responding to their prayers. HPs should display extra caution when approaching such patients about spiritual matters (but not avoid doing so).

In another case, a Christian physician asked a patient who was a Jehovah's Witness if the patient would like to pray with him. The patient said no. When the physician gently explored why this religious patient did not want prayer, she said that the physician's use of the word "God" instead of Jehovah in the prayer would have been offensive to her. Again, HPs must carefully explore the patient's religious background and find out what kind of a prayer would be most supportive for a given situation, and only if the patient wants prayer.

A fourth case, which occurred in a hospital in Fort Worth, involved a social worker. A medical patient was in the ICU after surgery and had not yet become fully conscious. The social worker at the hospital placed a "tract" (pamphlet encouraging Christian conversion) on the bedside table of the patient. The patient's family, who were Jehovah's Witnesses, saw the pamphlet when visiting the patient. Upset by this, they sued the social worker and the hospital. This case emphasizes the need to always be patient centered when raising and addressing spiritual issues in medical settings. It is the patient's religious or spiritual beliefs that are to be supported, not the beliefs of the HP.

Below is a list of other negative consequences that are at least theoretically possible:

- A religious patient is offended because the HP is of a different religious background and the spiritual history is not tailored to the patient's religious faith.
- The patient's family is not of the same religious background as the patient or the HP, and is offended by the HP's supporting the patient's religious beliefs or praying with the patient.

• A religious patient feels challenged because his religious beliefs are not respected during the spiritual history, or because the HP deals with his beliefs in a flippant manner.

• A nonreligious patient is upset because the HP is asking questions that hit a sensitive area in her life; she questions the HP's intentions and resents the implication that she is not religious "enough."

• Bringing up spiritual issues at times of serious illness creates undue anxiety in the patient, as this starts him thinking about whether the illness might be a punishment from God or what might happen to him after he dies.

• An unintended message is sent to the patient that she is nearing death and that nothing more can be done, creating anxiety and causing the patient to lose hope and give up.

• Spiritual issues come up that the HP is unprepared to handle or doesn't have time to address, and there are no clergy readily available to assist.

• After the spiritual history, the patient asks the HP what his or her religious beliefs are, and the HP does not feel comfortable sharing that information with the patient.

These concerns often scare HPs away from addressing spiritual issues with patients. How might the HP respond to each of the negative consequences described above? Here are some possible responses or ways of avoiding such situations.

A religious patient is offended because the HP is of a different religious background and the spiritual assessment is not tailored to the patient's religious faith.

Response: Always determine the patient's religious tradition first, and then tailor the spiritual history to that faith tradition. If the HP is unfamiliar with the faith tradition, then questions should be quite general without probing and, if necessary, either a professional chaplain consulted or the patient asked if he or she would like to speak with someone from his or her faith about any spiritual issues.

The patient's family is not of the same religious background as the HP or the patient, and is offended by the HP's supporting the patient's religious beliefs or praying with the patient.

Response: The HP's primary responsibility is always to the patient. Sometimes this needs to be gently explained to family members, who may or may not be satisfied by this response. In situations where religious conflict is possible, always get the chaplain's input.

A religious patient feels challenged because his religious beliefs are not respected during the spiritual assessment, or because the HP deals with his beliefs in a flippant manner.

Response: HPs should always show respect for the patient's religious beliefs, even when they conflict with recommended medical treatments. Efforts should be made to understand those beliefs, treat them seriously, and determine how they might influence the patient's coping with illness or medical decisions.

A nonreligious patient is upset because the HP is asking questions that hit a sensitive area in her life; she questions the HP's intentions and resents the implication that she is not religious "enough."

Response: The HP should always explain that a spiritual history is being conducted on all patients and is simply a matter of routine in order to fulfill the JCAHO requirement. As soon as the HP determines that the patient is not religious, the spiritual history ends, and this is documented in the medical record. Further questions should then be redirected towards determining what resources the patient relies on to cope with illness, and these resources then supported and made available to the patient as possible.

Bringing up spiritual issues at times of serious illness creates undue anxiety in the patient, as this starts him thinking about whether the illness might be a punishment from God or what might happen to him after he dies.

Response: The HP should be alert for such reactions, which may be reduced by proper preparation of the patient beforehand but may not be entirely avoidable. Before taking a spiritual history, explain to the patient that the hospital is trying to be sensitive to patients who have spiritual needs that might influence their health care and identify those who might want to speak with a chaplain.

An unintended message is sent to the patient that she is nearing death and that nothing more can be done, creating anxiety and causing the patient to lose hope and give up.

Response: Always prepare the patient before taking a spiritual history. Explain that these questions are simply a matter of routine, are asked of all patients, and have nothing to do with how serious the patient's medical condition is.

Spiritual issues come up that the HP is unprepared to handle or doesn't have time to address, and there are no clergy readily available to assist.

Response: Emphasize to the patient that the HP recognizes the seriousness of these spiritual concerns, that the HP will now contact someone who can address the concerns in a sensitive and professional way, and that the HP will follow up with the patient afterward to be sure that person adequately addressed his or her spiritual needs.

After the spiritual history, the patient asks the HP what his or her religious beliefs are, and the HP does not feel comfortable sharing that information with the patient.

Response: HPs are not obligated to share their personal religious beliefs with patients. If possible, though, try to avoid being defensive or rejecting when responding to such questions. Redirecting the conversation to medical matters may be one way to handle such situations. Alternatively, the HP may respond by emphasizing that he or she understands and appreciates how important the patient's religious beliefs are and will always honor and respect those beliefs. Often, quite simple and vague answers will satisfy the patient (i.e., "I'm Christian," or "I believe in God," or "I believe in a power greater than humans," etc.).

There is no systematic research examining how often such negative consequences actually occur. However, it appears that in both clinical practice and research studies, the overall positive consequences of addressing spiritual issues far outweigh the negative ones, both in frequency and impact.

SUMMARY AND CONCLUSIONS

Addressing spiritual issues as part of patient care—taking a brief spiritual history, supporting the patient's beliefs, validating religious distress, making appropriate pastoral care referrals, and, in carefully selected cases, even praying with patients—may have a number of potential benefits. It may also have negative consequences for both patient and HP if done without sensitivity, respect, or common sense. On the one hand, addressing spiritual issues may enhance the patient's ability to cope with illness, improve the HP-patient relationship, boost compliance with and belief in the treatment, and increase support and monitoring in the community, thereby improving satisfaction with care and speeding recovery from illness; and from the HP's side, practicing whole-person health care may reap deep rewards, leading to greater fulfillment and a return of idealism previously lost. On the other hand, when HPs address spiritual issues without sensitivity and respect, the results can be disastrous—leading to patient and family dissatisfaction and even expensive litigation.

CHAPTER 5

BOUNDARIES AND BARRIERS

This chapter explores the duties of the HP and the limitations in that role as it applies to addressing the spiritual needs of patients. What ethical boundaries should not be crossed? When is informed consent required? Are there gray areas that must be addressed on a case-by-case basis? Are there other pitfalls to avoid and dangers to be alert for when addressing spiritual issues? I explore further here some of the resistances, fears, and concerns that HPs have about bringing up religious or spiritual issues with patients. Although much of the content of this chapter is directed toward physicians, these principles apply in one way or another to all HPs.

HEALTH PROFESSIONAL'S ROLE

Most jobs have a job description. What are the responsibilities of the HP? Widely known medical ethicist and practicing physician Edmund Pelligrino has written extensively for more than two decades on the role of the physician, and these words of wisdom also apply to other health profession-als.[1] He has developed a model that relies on four words: profes-sion, patient, compassion, and consent. By "profession," he means the obligation to be competent and skillful in practice, the need to place the well-being of patients above self-interest, and the vol-untary manner in which HPs offer their skills to the patient who needs them. By "patient," Pelligrino means that the person seek-ing medical care is suffering and in a vulnerable position, and that the HP has the power to influence the patient's decisions and life. By "compassion," he means that the HP is called to suffer with the patient in sharing the existential situation the patient is in (which suggests a spiritual role as well). By "consent," he emphasizes that the HP-patient relationship is based on a freely given, informed consent by both parties involved, and that this consent should be made in the absence of pressure or force by one over the other.

In addition to these guidelines for HP-patient interactions, codes or oaths that HPs often take on graduating from their train-ing describe what respected HPs historically have believed the role of the HP to be. Among the most famous of these codes are the Hippocratic Oath and the oath of Maimonides. Written around the fifth century BC by the influential Greek physician Hippocrates, the original oath reads as follows:[2]

> I swear by Apollo the physician, by Aesculapius, Hygeia, and Pan-acea, and I take to witness all the gods, all the goddesses, to keep according to my ability and my judgment the following oath: To consider dear to me as my parents him who taught me this art; to live in common with him and if necessary to share my goods with him; to look upon his children as my own brothers, to teach them this art if they so desire without fee or written promise; to impart to my sons and the sons of the master who taught me and the dis-ciples who have enrolled themselves and have agreed to the rules of the profession, but to these alone, the precepts and the instruc-

tion. I will prescribe regimen for the good of my patients according to my ability and my judgment and never do harm to anyone. To please no one will I prescribe a deadly drug, nor give advice which may cause his death. Nor will I give a woman a pessary to procure abortion. But I will preserve the purity of my life and my art. I will not cut for stone, even for patients in whom the disease is manifest; I will leave this operation to be performed by practitioners [specialists in this art]. In every house where I come I will enter only for the good of my patients, keeping myself far from all intentional ill-doing and all seduction, and especially from the pleasures of love with women or with men, be they free or slaves. All that may come to my knowledge in the exercise of my profession or outside of my profession or in daily commerce with men, which ought not to be spread abroad, I will keep secret and will never reveal. If I keep this oath faithfully, may I enjoy my life and practice my art, respected by all men and in all times; but if I swerve from it or violate it, may the reverse be my lot.

Allan Butler, a physician from Vineyard Haven, Massachusetts, provides us with this updated version of the Hippocratic Oath in an article published in the *New England Journal of Medicine*:

We physicians shall re-emphasize as basic to our profession the rational ethical principal of minimizing suffering. In the course of our training and practice let us not be so intrigued with the intellectual satisfactions of understanding disease that we forget the priority of this humanitarian principle and the consideration of patients as people. In our role as specialists, let us have empathy with our patients. May we seek the potentialities of physical, mental and *spiritual* [emphasis added] health of each person and family and of society. We shall try new therapy or procedures only in fields in which we are experts and in consultation with other experts and only in which, in the opinion of experts, the possible benefit to the patient outweighs the possible risk. As the effectiveness of our services improves, let us fulfill our mounting responsibility to increase their availability. As the cost of our increasingly effective services rises, let us try to deliver them with increasing efficiency. Pretense will not enter our practice. Inability to help many of our patients will evoke our humility. Their suffering will be attended with compassion. In our reverence for life, let us not confound our minimization of suffering by compounding it in prolonging life nor give priority to quantity rather than quality of life. In practicing ethical principles beneficial to man, may we do unto others as we would that they do unto us, our children and man's genetic heritage.[3]

Moses Maimonides, who lived from AD 1135 to 1204, was perhaps the most important Jewish philosopher of the Middle Ages. Born in the Spanish city of Córdoba, Maimonides fled from southern Spain to Cairo because of rising anti-Semitism in Spain. In Cairo, Maimonides worked as a physician, and also became a scholar of Jewish law and a philosopher. He is responsible for composing the following oath that bears his name:

> The eternal Providence has appointed me to watch over the life and health of Thy creatures. May the love for my art actuate me at all time; may neither avarice nor miserliness, nor thirst for glory or for a great reputation engage my mind; for the enemies of truth and philanthropy could easily deceive me and make me forgetful of my lofty aim of doing good to Thy children. May I never see in the patient anything but a fellow creature in pain. Grant me the strength, time and opportunity always to correct what I have acquired, always to extend its domain; for knowledge is immense and the spirit of man can extend indefinitely to enrich itself daily with new requirements. Today he can discover his errors of yesterday and tomorrow he can obtain a new light on what he thinks himself sure of today. Oh, God, Thou has appointed me to watch over the life and death of Thy creatures; here am I ready for my vocation and now I turn unto my calling.[4]

Pelligrino's four words and these oaths emphasize that the responsibilities of the HP go beyond that of a typical employee or of a highly skilled technician. They emphasize that taking care of patients is more like a sacred, holy calling than anything else, and that the duty of the HP is to relieve the suffering of patients with expertise and compassion. They also emphasize that the relationship between HP and patient is a free one, entered into by mutual consent without coercion, and that the HP is in a position of power over the patient, who is vulnerable to the influence of the HP. Butler's version of the Hippocratic oath includes the responsibility of the HP for the health of the whole person— physical, mental, and spiritual. What, then, do these duties of the HP tell us about the limitations of that role and the boundaries that must be observed when addressing the spiritual needs of patients?

ROLE LIMITATIONS

HPs without pastoral training are limited in their level of expertise. HPs are not clergypersons, nor are they professional healthcare chaplains who have been trained to help patients resolve complex spiritual problems related to physical or emotional illness. HPs vary widely in religious background and in knowledge of the religious beliefs and practices of their patients, and many are unfamiliar with religious explanations for illness even in their own religious traditions. Thus, while any HP can take a spiritual history in a respectful manner, learning about the patient's religious beliefs, religious resources, and religious struggles in the face of illness (as a part of a duty to assess the whole patient), most HPs cannot provide theological explanations that adequately meet the spiritual needs of sick patients.

Similarly, any HP can support the beliefs the patient identifies as helpful and comforting, but few HPs have the expertise to provide advice on what beliefs or practices are most helpful for a particular patient, with a particular illness, in a particular religious belief system. Some HPs may choose to honor the request to pray with a patient and, if specific conditions are met, even initiate a simple prayer in carefully selected cases. However, most HPs do not have the training to advise patients on what to pray for, how to pray, or when or how often to pray, even if asked by patients.

NEED FOR CONSENT

Taking a brief screening spiritual history as part of the social history or supporting the patient's own religious beliefs does not require detailed discussion and consent beforehand. This is simply part of the comprehensive assessment and support of the whole person that is implied when the patient seeks the HP for treatment of a medical condition. Doing anything beyond simple screening and support, however, requires the fully informed and uncoerced consent of the patient. Because the patient is in a vulnerable position with respect to the HP, the obtaining of uncoerced consent to a spiritual intervention can be very difficult—not impossible, but difficult. Initiating prayer with patients, for example, should take place only when the HP knows beyond any doubt that the patient would welcome such a suggestion. This is true simply because the patient is not in a position to refuse the HP (who makes critical decisions about medical treatments that will influence the patient's life). Furthermore, the patient doesn't have the power to give consent to allow the HP to provide in-depth spiritual advice or deal with complex spiritual issues unless that HP has the training and expertise to provide such counseling.

The HP also needs to obtain consent before asking a chaplain or pastoral counselor to see the patient. This is particularly true in hospital settings. Likewise, before discussing a patient's case with the patient's clergy, parish nurse, or member of the patient's religious congregation, the HP must obtain consent from the patient. The patient should fully control and approve any communications between the HP and chaplain, clergy, or others members of the religious community. Except in emergency situations, the same would be true for referral of the patient to any other medical specialist or consultant, that is, there is a need to explain the reason for the consultation to the patient and seek his or her permission. Nevertheless, in some hospital settings, the chaplain may be viewed as part of the hospital staff that provides care to the patient—just like nurses. In that case, an argument could be made that consent to see a chaplain may not be needed prior to referral. Be aware that opinions vary on this issue, and it is probably wise to at least let the patient know prior to chaplain referral.

BOUNDARIES

Boundaries refer to the limitations in the role of the HP and the limitations in the role of the patient. Boundaries are necessary so that the HP can be as objective as possible when caring for the patient and making decisions about treatment. Objectivity is important so that emotional issues do not cloud medical judgments. Boundaries are also necessary from the patient's side to limit the expectations that patients place on their HPs.

Limitations in HP boundaries are more or less set within a given health care specialty, although they do vary across specialties. As pointed out earlier, boundaries set for a psychiatrist, psychologist, or psychiatric nurse are narrower than those for other HPs. The reason is that these mental health (MH) professionals treat patients who are often unsure of their own identity and have difficulty recognizing their boundaries as patients. This is especially true for patients with personality disorders (borderline personality disorder being the most severe). If MH professionals cross over boundaries, or fail to hold patients accountable for overstepping their boundaries, then the therapeutic relationship may become altered so that effective treatment becomes impossible. See chapter 11 for further discussion of the unique role of MH professionals and boundary issues related to that role.

Boundaries between surgeons and patients are also important to maintain, although to a lesser degree than between psychiatrists and patients. If the surgeon is operating on a good friend, this could increase his or her stress during the operation. For that reason, the surgeon tries to remain as objective as possible in his or her feelings toward the patient in order to reduce the risk of surgical error. Boundaries between primary care physician (family physician, pediatrician, or internist) and patient are also necessary, although probably to a lesser degree than for a surgeon or a psychiatrist, and to a lesser degree still for a medical nurse or a social worker than for a primary care physician. Again, when the role of the HP is purely supportive, boundary issues can be relaxed (but again, not totally dismissed).

Spiritual assessment and support do not typically threaten boundaries. An exception may be when the MH professional is doing insight-oriented therapy, where supporting or encouraging religious beliefs would not be proper. Boundaries become more of an issue when an HP decides to pray with a patient or offer spiritual advice. Because religion is such an intensely emotional and deeply personal area (for both patients and HPs), it is more difficult to maintain objectivity after such spiritual interventions—not impossible, but more difficult. Again, there is less risk for primary care physicians, medical nurses, medical social workers, and rehabilitation therapists when they are dealing with patients in stressful medical circumstances, where providing emotional support is the primary objective. Being aware of the dangers of over-involvement and making efforts to maintain professional boundaries, however, will help HPs regardless of specialty to increase their therapeutic effectiveness.

GRAY AREAS

It is essential to keep in mind that there will always be gray areas in terms of boundaries that must be dealt with on a case-by-case basis. For example, consider the case of an older male patient whom we will call Bill. Bill has several chronic health problems, lives alone, and has become increasingly depressed and socially isolated since his wife died two years ago. Social history uncovers that Bill has no close family members in the area. A spiritual history taken by an HP reveals that Bill is quite religious and used to be very active in his church. Because of a conflict with pastoral staff five years ago, however, he stopped attending services and has not returned. He says that he regrets this and misses the friends he had at church. Sensing that Bill might have a spiritual problem, the HP asks if he would like a referral to see a pastoral counselor. Bill declines, saying that he doesn't want to talk with any clergy. The HP prescribes an antidepressant and provides a referral for secular psychotherapy (which Bill also refuses).

When Bill returns for his follow-up appointment a month later, the HP notes that while his mood has improved, he remains socially withdrawn. At the end of the visit, he gently asks Bill what happened five years ago when he stopped attending services. With great emotion, the patient recalls the angry discussion he had with the music leader about the type of music played in church. The HP listens attentively for about five minutes. At the end, he suggests that Bill consider reconnecting with his former church or find another one. When the patient returns a month later, his depression is much improved. Bill tells the HP that he has attended church services at his former church for the past two weeks and is reconnecting with many old friends.

In this case, the HP identified a spiritual need by taking a spiritual history. Since the spiritual problem appeared complex, he tried to refer the patient to a religious professional. Seeing the need for socialization, and realizing that the patient would not see a pastoral counselor or any counselor for that matter, the HP decided to address the spiritual problem by carefully exploring a little further and then suggesting that he return to church. By taking a few minutes to listen to the patient describe the problem in greater detail, the HP helped him work through it. Addressing the spiritual problem and suggesting a solution went beyond the HP's area of expertise. However, the HP tried the more appropriate route (referral) first, and only when that avenue was blocked, he decided to take on the problem himself. Furthermore, by suggesting Bill return to attending church services, the HP was not introducing or recommending anything new to Bill, since the spiritual history revealed that this had once been a very important area of his life. While the case had a good outcome because Bill responded well to the spiritual intervention, many other outcomes are also possible.

Real situations are always more complex and complicated than can be addressed by rigidly applying a set of rules. The guidelines presented above, however, provide a framework that will help guide HPs in different situations and maximize positive outcomes.

THE POWER OF CARING

The above text has emphasized the importance of role limitations, the maintenance of relationship boundaries between HP and patient, and the need to be flexible in terms of applying these basic guidelines. This discussion would be incomplete, however, without pointing out that sometimes HPs need to take risks. We often deal with patients who are going through incredibly difficult life circumstances, who are lonely, isolated, and carrying tremendous physical and psychological burdens. They come to us for help, often desperate and with nowhere else to go. Sometimes there is no other way to help them but to get involved in their lives, start to really care as a friend, and communicate that to them. This involves self-sacrifice and going beyond the call of duty, taking a risk that will possibly compromise the HP's objectivity in medical decision making. It is a risk taken out of kindness and compassion. It is a risk that some of the best HPs take all the time.

OTHER PITFALLS AND DANGERS

Most problems that result from addressing spiritual issues occur because the HP either steps beyond the boundaries of competency by addressing issues that lie in the expertise of professional religious caregivers or does not follow up on spiritual needs to ensure that they are adequately addressed. The responsibility of the HP lies in identifying spiritual needs and orchestrating resources to meet those needs. If time is a problem, and delegating that responsibility to others becomes necessary, then the HP must always follow up with the patient to ensure that resources were mobilized to meet the need.

Assuming a patient is religious or has a good relationship with his religious community, without taking an adequate spiritual history, is a pitfall to be avoided. This is particularly true if a spiritual intervention (such as referral to a chaplain, discussion with the patient's clergyperson, or initiation of prayer) is considered.

Such mistakes are usually made during crisis situations either in the emergency room or in the hospital, when there is little time for assessment. The problem is failure to obtain consent because of lack of adequate information. It takes only a moment to check with the patient or a family member about the patient's spiritual orientation and whether a spiritual intervention would be appreciated or best avoided.

Providing spiritual advice to patients is another potential pitfall. When there are similarities in religious background, the HP may be tempted to resolve ideological problems for patients by providing them with correct religious views. This can often deteriorate into religious debates or can overextend the HP into a position that can bring attack or devaluation by the patient. Asking questions to help patients clarify their thinking about a spiritual problem is always better than giving advice.

When addressing spiritual issues, HPs must also be aware of how their own religious beliefs can interfere with their ability to evaluate a situation objectively.[5] For example, an HP with conservative religious views may be tempted to impose those views on a patient seeking an abortion, having premarital sex, or involved in an adulterous relationship outside of marriage or in a homosexual affair. Such behaviors may evoke feelings of disdain or disgust in religious HPs toward such patients, compromising their ability to meet the patients' health care needs effectively. In the same way, nonreligious HPs may dismiss the conservative religious views of patients as regressive or Victorian, and allow their personal religious views to influence the quality of care that they deliver. HPs must constantly be on guard for such "countertransference" reactions within themselves.

BARRIERS AND FEARS

While it is true that HPs must proceed with caution and sensitivity when addressing spiritual issues, many don't even try to do so because of personal resistance, fears, or unjustified concerns about delving into this area. I have already reviewed numerous cautions, pitfalls, and dangers so that HPs will be fully prepared to address spiritual issues in an effective manner, equipped to handle or avoid problems that may come up during the process. This should not, however, frighten anyone away—regardless of specialty—from doing a spiritual history, referring to pastoral care specialists, and, in rare instances, compassionately addressing spiritual issues as they arise.

A number of barriers, both real and attitudinal, keep HPs from assessing spiritual issues in clinical practice. These include lack of knowledge, lack of training, lack of time, concerns about projecting beliefs onto patients, uncertainty on how to address spiritual issues raised by patients, and especially, personal discomfort when HPs are not religious or spiritual themselves.[6] Most of this research has been done on physicians, although it likely applies to other HPs as well.

Lack of Knowledge. Many HPs are not aware of how important religious beliefs and practices are to sick patients, nor do they know about the research that links religious practices to better coping and better health. Because HPs tend to be somewhat less religious than their patients,[7] they often don't realize that patients—particularly religious patients—might want them to address spiritual issues or might have religious beliefs that could affect their medical decisions. Finally, most HPs are not aware of the potential benefits of addressing spiritual issues, in terms of the HP-patient relationship and even the course of the medical illness, based on a rapidly growing research base connecting religion and health.

Lack of Training. Although over 100 of the 141 medical schools in the United States now have either elective or required courses on religion/spirituality and medicine, most physicians in practice have no training in this regard. Furthermore, many students graduating from medical schools today don't either, since about one-third of these courses are elective and have small attendance. Many physicians don't know how to take a spiritual history, don't know when to do it, and don't know what to do if spiritual needs come up during the evaluation. Unfortunately, many are also perfectly content practicing medicine exactly as they have been doing and don't want the additional burden of having to ask patients about their spiritual beliefs. Studies show, however, that even a single hour and a half or two-hour workshop on spirituality and medicine can make a significant difference in knowledge and attitudes of medical students and residents.[8]

Lack of Time. In the late 1990s, a study of 170 Missouri family physicians found that 71 percent indicated lack of time as a barrier to addressing spiritual issues.[9] Lack of time ranked number one among fourteen barriers that were asked about, and lack of training or experience in taking a spiritual history was number two (nearly 60%). According to a more recent survey in the same geographic location,[10] however, lack of time was *not* a significant predictor of physicians' addressing spiritual issues. Only 26 percent indicated that they did not have time to discuss religious issues with patients. Furthermore, in Curlin and colleagues' most recent study of a national sample of 1,144 physicians of all specialties, less than half (48%) indicated that lack of time was a major barrier to discussing religious or spiritual matters with patients.[11] Interestingly, those physicians who indicated lack of time as a barrier were actually *more likely* to discuss R/S issues with patients compared to other physicians. Although time is short in the HP-patient encounter, asking a couple of questions about how the patient is doing spiritually does not take much time (less than five minutes and more likely only two or three minutes). If spiritual needs are identified, a referral to a chaplain or pastoral counselor is easily done. Studies have shown that people with emotional problems would rather see a clergyperson than a counselor, psychologist, or a psychiatrist.[12]

Discomfort with the Subject. One of the most common reasons why HPs do not inquire about spiritual issues is interpersonal discomfort. In a survey of predictors of proactive religious inquiry by physicians,[13] investigators found that interpersonal discomfort (i.e., responding yes to the statement "I am uncomfortable addressing religious issues with patients") was the only independent predictor of physician inquiry. Other significant predictors in the uncontrolled analysis (physician specialty, not relevant to health, not in job description) all lost their significance when interpersonal discomfort was added to the model. Likewise, in the Curlin and colleagues' study of 1,144 randomly sampled U.S. physicians, lack of comfort was the only variable in multivariate analyses that predicted lower rates of physician inquiry about R/S issues; physicians who reported lack of comfort were 40 percent less likely to address R/S issues.[14] Lack of comfort is hardly a good reason to avoid asking about an important area of the patient's life that is so closely linked with psychological and physical health and decisions about medical care. As expected in that study, family physicians and internists (primary care physicians) were more likely than neurologists and surgeons to inquire about spiritual issues.

Fear of Imposing Religious Views or Offending Patients. While this is often talked about as a concern, most physicians in at least one study did not agree that this was a good reason for not discussing religious issues with patients. In the Chibnall and Brooks study, 75 percent of physicians disagreed with the statement, "Because physicians may impose their religious views on patients, physicians should not discuss religious issues with them."[15] Although concern about offending patients is a worry for many HPs, it is not the most common concern. In the Curlin study discussed above, only a minority of physicians indicated that concern about offending patients was a barrier to their discussing R/S issues.

Knowledge about Religion not Relevant to Medical Care. In the mid-1980s, the majority of physicians did not believe that religious beliefs or practices of patients had an impact on physical health or medical outcomes.[16] That view, however, is changing. In the Chibnall and Brooks study conducted in 2001, 63 percent of physicians indicated that the patient's religiousness affects health. In the same study, 64 percent of physicians agreed with the statement, "Physician acknowledgment and support of patient religious values can improve the process and outcome of healthcare provision"; only 8 percent disagreed with that statement.[17] More recently, Monroe and colleagues found that 85 percent of physicians indicated that the doctor should be aware of the patient's R/S beliefs[18] and, among family physicians, Ellis and colleagues found that 96 percent indicated that spiritual well-being is an important component of health.[19]

Not in My Job Description. In a random sample of 160 Illinois family physicians, 69 percent disagreed with a statement indicating that only clergy should address religious issues.[20] In a study of 115 active members of the Vermont Academy of Family Physicians, the majority believed that the physician has a right (89%)

and the responsibility (52%) to inquire about religious factors in patient care.[21] The Chibnall and Brooks study also found that the majority of physicians rejected the notion that addressing religious issues was not in their job description.

OVERCOMING BARRIERS

Lack of knowledge of religion's effects on health and lack of training on how and when to address religious or spiritual issues is easily rectified by exposing HPs to research on religion and health and providing some training. Fear of imposing the HP's religious beliefs on patients does not appear to be a major issue, and the majority of physicians believe that it is both appropriate and responsible for physicians to address spiritual issues as part of patient care. What appears to be the major impediment to HP inquiry about religious issues is *personal discomfort* with the topic. Discomfort with the topic, however, correlates strongly with physician religiosity, and religious physicians indicate much greater comfort with discussing such issues than do less religious physicians.[22] Although making physicians more religious is not either an ethical or a practical goal, training on the importance of addressing these issues and actual practice doing it can help reduce the discomfort

Inadequate time is still a real barrier to addressing religious issues, despite Chibnall and Brooks's report that only 24 percent of physicians gave it as an excuse for not doing so. While not every patient needs spiritual screening on every visit, it still takes time to find out about a patient's spiritual history and it takes time to be supportive and to address spiritual issues that may come up. Physicians and other HPs need to decide whether this area is important enough to take the extra time when the

situation calls for it. As health care systems learn about the connection between religion and health, and if future studies demonstrate that addressing spiritual needs improves health outcomes,
reduces service use, and improves patient satisfaction, then perhaps HPs and health care systems will be compensated for the
extra time spent inquiring about these issues, a practice that, in
the long run, may result in better care and lower cost.

SUMMARY AND CONCLUSIONS

It is important to understand the roles and responsibilities of HPs,
as well as the limitations on how far they should go in addressing
spiritual issues. Obtaining patient consent is essential, as is maintaining HP boundaries as they apply to taking a spiritual history,
supporting religious beliefs, praying with patients, or referring to
clergy. Gray areas must be acknowledged in order to maintain
flexibility in these matters and to prevent a rigid adherence to
boundaries. Other pitfalls and dangers of HP inquiry about spiritual issues need to be recognized and avoided. Finally, HPs must
examine and overcome concerns and discomforts over talking
about spirituality with patients.

CHAPTER 6

WHEN RELIGION (OR SPIRITUALITY) IS HARMFUL

What about the negative effects of religion or spirituality on health? Recent articles by psychologist Richard P. Sloan in the *Lancet*[1] and the *New England Journal of Medicine*[2] have challenged the research linking religion and health as weak and inconsistent and have emphasized the harm that can result when HPs address spiritual issues. "Do no harm" (from the Hippocratic Oath) is perhaps the most important rule in medical ethics. Are there times when religious or spiritual beliefs can actually interfere with medical care, lead to health problems, or worsen disease outcomes? What are some examples and how often this occurs? How can clinicians handle such situations in a sensitive, thoughtful, and effective manner? What about HPs actually causing harm by inquiring about R/S issues?

NEGATIVE EFFECTS OF RELIGION

Obviously not all of the effects of religion on health are positive, and it is important for HPs to be aware of times when R/S beliefs may worsen health problems or conflict with appropriate medical care. Conventional wisdom proves that religion has been used to justify all sorts of negative behaviors throughout history. Religion can cause people to be judgmental and lead to alienation or exclusion of those not playing "by the rules." Religion may become so rigid and inflexible that it becomes excessively restricting and limiting. Religion may encourage magical thinking as people pray for and expect physical healing as if God were a giant genie at the beck and call of every human whim. Then, if physical healing does not come immediately, the person may be disappointed and disheartened, claiming that the prayer was not answered and that God does not care, or, worse, that the illness was sent by an angry, vengeful God as a punishment. These uses of religion are not uncommon in health care settings, causing distress and potentially have a negative impact on illness and its response to treatment.

Devout religious involvement may also lead to more subtle psychological and social strains that can influence the well-being of patients and family members. These include interpersonal strains, inner struggles to believe, and problems with virtuous strivings.[3] Interpersonal strains result from religious disagreements and negative attitudes towards other religious groups. Conversion to a different religious group (from Christian to Buddhist, or from Catholic to evangelical Christian, for example) may cause disharmony, anger, and pain to other family members, close friends, and patients themselves. Another example is when one spouse comes from a different religion than the other, with resulting arguments over leadership roles, the raising of children, ways of spending time together, establishment of family traditions, and financial matters, often based on differing religious views. Conflict may also arise when a person is so involved in church activities that he or she neglects a spouse, children, or other responsibilities around the home. This may lead to marital or family discord and deep-seated resentments that could adversely affect that person's mental health and family support when sick.

Inner struggles to believe may also create conflict. Nonbelievers may experience distress related to the dominant Judeo-Christian culture in which they live. Unable to logically and rationally endorse a religious belief system, they may nevertheless desire for life to have greater meaning (especially when sick and suffering) or to have greater support from their community (as members of faith communities might have). Furthermore, many nonbelievers are not strict atheists, may wonder about whether there is some truth in religion, and may fear that they have missed something important.

Finally, patients may experience distress over virtuous strivings. Religious people strive to better themselves in ways prescribed by their religious group. This may involve a lifestyle that includes self-sacrifice, nonparticipation in certain kinds of activities, or avoidance of certain kinds of people. Such a lifestyle may alienate them from their social group or from the culture at large. This may create inner conflict over desires to be true to religious teachings and yet also to be approved and included by others. Likewise, religious people may have high values that they are trying to live by (sexual morality, honesty, generosity, forgiveness, humility, or kindness) and may often fail to live up to such high standards, resulting in feelings of guilt, self-condemnation, and discouragement. Thus, psychological, social, and spiritual strains may result from devout religious involvement or lack thereof.

These may create inner conflicts and struggles that can influence mental health and medical outcomes.

Equally as worrisome, religion may be used *instead of* medical care. Members of certain fundamentalist religious sects may fail to seek prenatal or obstetrical care on religious grounds, greatly increasing the risk of infant and maternal mortality (e.g., Faith Assembly in Indiana).[4] Active resistance against childhood vaccination occurs in a number of religious groups around the world and has resulted in outbreaks of polio,[5] rubella,[6] whooping cough,[7] and other infectious diseases,[8] although recent research indicates that religious exemptions to pertussis vaccination may not have as great an impact as other factors.[9]

Certain life-saving treatments may be avoided or discontinued on religious grounds. Jehovah's Witnesses may refuse life-saving blood products, and some Christian Scientists may avoid seeing HPs, relying on prayer instead. Patients may stop their medications after attending a healing service in order to "demonstrate their faith." This is done with the best of intentions and is completely logical within the particular belief system. Diabetics may stop their insulin, hypothyroid patients their thyroid hormone, asthmatics their bronchodilators, or epileptics their anti-seizure medications. Unfortunately, such decisions are usually followed by negative consequences[10] and the HP is left to pick up the pieces (often not knowing why the patient's condition has deteriorated). This is another reason patients need to feel free to talk to their HPs about spiritual matters.

FREQUENCY OF RELIGIOUS CONFLICTS

There are times, then, when religion conflicts with standard medical care and patients decide in favor of religion rather than risk being alienated from a belief system that gives their lives purpose, meaning, and hope (and perhaps being ostracized from their social group). But how often does this actually happen? Is this a common occurrence that HPs confront every day in their offices, or is this a relatively rare event that is the exception rather than the rule? Based on what we know from the existing research, conflicts between religion and medical treatments are not very common, but they do occur. When they occur, much attention is generated, ethics committees are convened, newspaper stories appear, and so on. Most of our patients are affiliated with traditional religious groups that maintain sensible policies when it comes to need for medical care, and research suggesting otherwise has often been methodologically unsound.

Consider Asser and Swan's 1998 report[11] in the prestigious medical journal *Pediatrics* that 172 children died between 1975 and 1995 from parental withholding of medical care on religious grounds. Investigators reported examples of children dying from food aspiration, cancer, pneumonia, meningitis, diabetes, asthma, and other treatable childhood illnesses. The 172 deaths were distributed across twenty-three denominations located in thirty-four states. Careful examination, however, revealed that 83 percent of the total fatalities came from five religious groups: fifty from Indiana (primarily from Faith Assembly, referred to above), sixteen from Pennsylvania (most from Faith Tabernacle), fifteen from Oklahoma and Colorado (mainly from Church of the First Born), five from End Time Ministries in South Dakota, and twenty-eight from members of Christian Science nationwide. These are hardly mainstream religious groups, and it is safe to say that the total national membership of all these religious groups combined makes up less than 1 percent of all Americans.

Furthermore, the methodology of Asser and Swan's study

makes it almost impossible to determine how often withholding of medical care from children on religious grounds actually occurs. Even the authors admit that "calculations of overall incidence and mortality rates are not possible in this study as the number of children in the group sampled is not available and the cases were collected in a *non-rigorous manner*" (p. 628). "Nonrigorous" means that most cases were collected over the previous fifteen years from newspaper articles, public documents, trial records, and personal communications obtained from the files of Swan's advocacy group, CHILD. Also, prediction of whether or not these children would have survived with medical care was based on the judgment of a single pediatrician (the study's lead author). The science in this study, then, was largely subjective, and the results and conclusions could have been strongly influenced by investigator bias.

There are also conflicts between religion and medicine that affect health care in adulthood. Many more examples, although almost no systematic research, exist for religious conflicts stemming from beliefs against receiving blood transfusions (Jehovah's Witnesses), seeking psychotherapy (certain fundamentalist Christian groups), or more subtle forms of noncompliance based on religious belief.[12] It is safe to say, though, that a large number of these problems could be avoided or minimized with better, more open communication between HPs and patients on spiritual issues.

HANDLING RELIGIOUS CONFLICTS

The key to handling situations where religious beliefs conflict with medical or psychiatric care is for the HP to enter into the worldview of the patient and attempt to understand the logic of the decision. There is always a clear reason in the mind of the patient for preferring religion to medicine when health or life is at stake, although this is often hidden from the HP. Unfortunately, the first and most natural response of many HPs is to be offended. The patient has chosen what appears to be a totally irrational treatment instead of the HP's scientifically proven therapy. This creates anger in the HP and sometimes rejection of the patient, leading to arguments and a breakdown of communication.

By entering into the patient's religious worldview, the HP will realize how serious a matter this is for the patient. For example, Jehovah's Witnesses refuse blood products because it is their religious conviction that God (Jehovah) will turn his back on anyone who receives blood transfusions. Rather than risk eternal damnation, Jehovah's Witnesses avoid blood transfusions for themselves and their children. To members of this religious denomination, a few more years spent suffering here on earth is not worth being ostracized from family and friends, and perhaps damnation for eternity after death. Within these patients' worldview, it makes absolutely no sense *not* to refuse blood products. Likewise, patients who attend a prayer service and have emotional experiences that convince them that they are healed pit their faith in God against faith in medicine. And faith in God who is with them every day may mean a lot more than faith in the HP whom they only see every six months.

What is important here is keeping lines of communication open between the HP and patient, regardless of what the patient decides. This may require that the HP accept religious patients' decisions to forego medical care and then medically follow them carefully. As long as patients feel that their beliefs and decisions are respected, they will be more likely to confide in an HP about these matters and turn back to medical treatments if things aren't working out.

Otherwise, patients may feel the need to defend themselves and will delay seeking medical help when they really need it.

In situations where religious beliefs conflict with medical care, sometimes it helps if the HP (after getting consent) speaks with the patient's clergy in order to obtain a better understanding of the patient's decision. This action will help the HP learn more about the religious belief system of the patient, will help to align the HP with the patient's religious authority, and will help clarify any misunderstandings that the patient may have concerning religious beliefs. Patients may sometimes use religious beliefs to justify actions that religious doctrines were never intended to justify. A brief conversation with the patient's clergy can often quickly identify such neurotic or defensive uses of religion and will enable the HP to enroll the clergyperson to help apply pressure on the patient to give them up.

HP INQUIRY CAUSING HARM

Does HP inquiry into religious or spiritual issues actually harm patients? Let's take a closer look at this claim.

Upsetting Patients. The argument here is that a brief screening spiritual history is upsetting to patients either because they don't expect it, because it is too personal, or because they are not religious. Patients come to see HPs to have health problems addressed, not their spiritual lives assessed. Religion is too personal to talk about in a medical setting, and HPs should not inquire about this area any more than they should inquire about a patient's choice of marital partner or decisions about personal finances. Finally, the patient who is not religious may become upset because HP inquiry about religious issues suggests that they are important and that failure to embrace them is abnormal or pathological.

Patients expect HPs to address issues related to their mental and physical health and their medical care. If religious issues had no bearing on health and had no effect on medical decisions, then inquiry about them would indeed go beyond the professional duty of the HP. Because of the significant role that religious or spiritual beliefs play in all these areas, however, it is important for HPs to know about them. HPs inquire into many personal aspects of patients' lives because those areas affect the patient's health or medical care. As part of the social history, it is imperative that HPs inquire about the marital status of patients, how many children they have, the kinds of supports they have in the community, and their financial status—each of which can affect the support the patient will receive at home and in the community and the likelihood that they will comply with medical treatment and receive adequate monitoring. HPs do not devalue patients who are single, without friends, or who are poor, but they do need to know about these conditions because of the potential relationship to health and the kind of support the patients will have once they leave the hospital or doctor's office. HPs also inquire about and make recommendations concerning many very private areas in patients' lives *if they are related to health*. This includes genetic counseling for those with genetic disorders who are planning to marry, sexual counseling for those with multiple sexual partners at risk for STDs, and counseling about health habits such as eating, smoking, drinking, and other private behaviors, all of which are deeply personal. Because of their relationships to health, they are within the domain of the HP's responsibility. The intention and purpose of such inquiries is not to promote religion, but to promote health and well-being. This is the entire purpose of the screening spiritual history: improving the health of the patient—a secular goal and one for which HPs are responsible.

HP inquiry about the spiritual beliefs and practices of patients should not offend those without such beliefs if inquiry is done in a sensitive and respectful manner. As noted in chapter 2, if patients indicate that religious or spiritual beliefs are not important in their lives, then the spiritual history should end and the HP should simply go on to explore what factors provide meaning, purpose, and support. Religion is certainly not the only source of fulfillment for basic existential and psychological needs during illness. Such a transition from a religious focus to a nonreligious one should be done so smoothly and seamlessly that the nonreligious patient hardly notices it. If there is indication that the patient has religious conflicts or struggles, however, then these need to be brought out into the open, because they may worsen the course of the illness and adversely affect medical outcomes.[13] Again, the HPs focus is always on maintaining and maximizing the health of the patient.

There is systematic research that has examined how often patients are upset by spiritual inquiries. The OASIS study mentioned earlier involved 118 patients who were randomly (alternately) assigned to oncologists.[14] The OASIS spiritual history was pretty extensive, taking an average of 6.0 minutes to administer, and went beyond the brief screening spiritual history that is recommended in this book. The authors point out, "It is important to distinguish the conceptual framework of this approach from that of taking a medical or spiritual 'history'. . . Rather, the structure [of OASIS] is intended to facilitate communication between patient and physician and to empower the patient, if need be, to more fully consider his or her own issues and resources in this domain." Physicians indicated that forty-eight of fifty-four patients (89%) receiving the intervention appeared "quite comfortable" or "very comfortable."

When patients were asked immediately after the intervention how comfortable they felt discussing spiritual issues with their oncologist, 74 percent said quite or very comfortable, 15 percent said somewhat comfortable, and 11 percent said a little comfortable or not at all comfortable. When asked the same question about comfort level three weeks later, only 6 percent of patients indicated they felt a little or not at all comfortable. These findings are even more striking given the fact that half of the oncologists administering the intervention were non-Christians (Hindu and Sikh), while over 80 percent of patients in the study were Christian and an additional 15 percent had no affiliation. Thus, based on this study, only about one in ten patients is likely to feel uncomfortable when the HP inquires about spiritual matters, and even fewer are likely to feel that way if the spiritual history is briefer and more focused on acquiring information (rather than on intervening as in the OASIS study).

Inducing Guilt. It is common for patients to have existential questions about their illnesses, and many inquire "Why me?" when given a devastating diagnosis. A sick patient may feel that the medical illness is a punishment from God. Again, the logic is not terribly difficult to understand: If devout religious faith is related to better physical health and protection from disease, then illness must result from lack of it. "Linking religious activities and better health outcomes can be harmful to patients, who already must confront age-old folk wisdom that illness is due to their own moral failure."[15]

The fact that questions such as "Why me?" are so common and may affect health outcomes, if anything, makes it essential that these concerns be brought out into the open and addressed. This only further justifies HP inquiry about spiritual issues. Research has shown that patients who feel deserted or punished by God or who question God's power or love have an increased likelihood of dying compared to patients without such feelings.[16] While the HP may not be the best person to address complex spiritual issues like these, someone needs to. As indicated earlier, chaplains and pastoral counselors are trained to address such questions but need to be alerted to the problem. Many patients with these beliefs, however, are alienated from religion because of their negative feelings toward it and don't want to speak to clergy, leaving the HP as the choice of last resort.

There is also risk of inducing patient guilt when HPs inquire about religious or spiritual issues. However, HPs take such risks all the time when they inquire about *any* behaviors that are related to health status—whether it is smoking, exercise, or diet. If a patient has lung cancer, the HP is obligated to ask about smoking even if the question makes the patient feel guilty about having smoked. What HP would not ask about exercise and diet in an obese patient with coronary artery disease, taking the risk of making the patient feel guilty for living a sedentary life or eating too much?

In fact, all counseling with regard to health maintenance or disease prevention runs the risk of making patients feel guilty if they don't follow recommendations and end up sick. Even recommendations to participate in a support group can cause guilt in the person who remains reclusive and then develops a recurrence of disease. Does the fear of inducing guilt prevent HPs from making inquiries about these issues? No, it does not. Nor should it stop them from doing a brief spirituality history.

However, there is more to be said about inducing guilt in sick patients about not having enough faith. Even the tiniest amount of intelligence or common sense would demand that HPs not make patients feel bad because they are not religious enough.

Physical and mental illnesses have many causes—genetic, developmental, accidental, traumatic—that have nothing whatsoever to do with religion or faith. Even the most devoutly religious people end up getting sick and dying. Are not all the saints and martyrs now dead? It is often not until a person becomes sick, experiences tragedy, or goes through some period of great suffering that deep religious faith emerges out of the struggle. Consequently, those with the most advanced illness often end up being those who are the most spiritual. Thus, it is impossible and often completely wrong to conclude that a patient's poor physical health is due to lack of faith—and HPs should never imply this.

CAN "SPIRITUALITY" BE HARMFUL?

Although the word "spirituality" is almost always associated with something good in today's popular culture, spirituality may also be associated with harm just as religion can be. Nonbelievers may react in the same negative way to spirituality as they would to religion, not being able to readily distinguish between the two. While we academicians make fine distinctions between religion and spirituality, most of our patients don't really know the difference between the two, and often understand religion and spirituality as the same thing.

There are also beliefs about spirits, spiritual beings or spiritual forces that can induce psychological or even physical harm to people (as in voodoo or witchcraft). Belief in demonic or evil spirits may lead to great distress in patients from spiritual traditions in which such forces are emphasized and where there is belief that people can become inhabited by such spirits.

Spiritual practices such as transcendental meditation, mindfulness meditation, healing touch (involving "subtle energies"), acupuncture, or Reiki may at times be offered to Christian patients as part of alternative or complementary medicine programs. Such spiritual practices may be presented by practitioners with an almost evangelical zeal to patients who are desperate for help after allopathic medical treatments have failed. Patients from conservative Christian groups may know very little about such practices, which are rooted in Eastern or New Age religious traditions and may directly conflict with their Christian religious beliefs.

HPs not knowledgeable about or insensitive to conservative Christian beliefs may impose these foreign spiritual practices on patients without fully explaining their origins and without providing traditional Christian alternatives more consistent with patients' beliefs (such as prayer, visit with a chaplain, access to religious services or religious literature like the Bible). Devout Muslim patients may likewise be offended when spiritual practices rooted in Eastern or New Age religious traditions are offered to them. Although there is little research on how often this occurs, my sense is that such practices are not at all uncommon in alternative and complementary centers at many major hospitals and medical centers in the United States today.

SUMMARY AND CONCLUSIONS

Besides the many positive effects that religion or spirituality may have on health, they can also have negative effects. Believers (and nonbelievers) may experience subtle psychological, social, and spiritual strains related to religious beliefs that distress them, their family, and their support network. Religious beliefs cause patients to forego needed medical care, refuse life-saving procedures, and stop necessary medication—choosing faith instead of medicine. While this does not occur very often, when it does occur, it creates much stir and distress for all involved. HPs need to learn to respect the decisions that patients make based on their religious beliefs and not become offended or feel rejected. Instead, they should try to enter into a patient's religious world-view in order to better understand the logic of the decision. Only in this way can the door of communication be kept open between HPs and the religious patient. The claim that HP inquiry about religious or spiritual issues can cause harm by upsetting patients or inducing excessive guilt is one that should be taken seriously and should motivate HPs to obtain training in this area. Nevertheless, this claim is not so water tight or so well substantiated that it should prevent HPs from addressing an area that may be of vital importance to many patients' psychological, social, and physical health.

CHAPTER 7

CHAPLAINS AND PASTORAL CARE

This chapter is primarily devoted to HPs without religious training to help them better understand who the pastoral care specialists are and the unique roles that each play in meeting the spiritual needs of patients with health problems. Although most of this section is about professional healthcare chaplains, who are the primary experts in spiritual care for the sick, I also discuss what pastoral counselors and community clergy do.

PROFESSIONAL CHAPLAINS

There are approximately ten thousand chaplains in the United States in full-time practice or training programs who provide 10 to 15 million hours of counseling each year. The four largest chaplain organizations are the Association of Professional Chaplains (APC, 4,000 members), the National Association of Catholic Chaplains (NACC, 4,000 members), the Association of Clinical Pastoral Education (ACPE, 1,000 members), and the National Association of Jewish Chaplains (NAJC, 400 members). Other chaplain organizations include the American Protestant Correctional Chaplains Association, Chaplaincy Commission of New York Board of Rabbis, Council on Ministries in Specialized Settings, International Conference of Police Chaplains, National Conference on Ministry to the Armed Forces, and National Institute of Business and Industrial Chaplaincy. These organizations are responsible for setting standards for and certifying members as professional chaplains.[1]

The Association of Professional Chaplains (APC) had its origins in the Association of Protestant Hospital Chaplains (APHC), which had its first meetings in the 1940s and dates back even further to the 1930s, when Russell Dicks and Richard Cabot (a physician) coauthored the classic book, *The Art of Ministering to the Sick.* In 1968, APHC was renamed the American College of Chaplains, and its membership grew rapidly. In the 1980s, the College of Chaplains and the Association of Mental Health Chaplains (AMHC) received support from the Commission for Hospital Accreditation to establish standards for chaplaincy. Also about this time, Medicare agreed to provide reimbursement to hospitals for chaplain services. In 1998, the College of Chaplains and AMHC merged to form the APC. The APC describes itself as "an interfaith professional pastoral care association of providers of pastoral care endorsed by faith groups to serve persons in physical, spiritual, or mental need in diverse settings throughout the world."[2] APC has a code of professional ethics, establishes standards of care, and seeks to identify "best practices" that are published in its journals, newsletter, and Web site.

The National Association of Catholic Chaplains (NACC) was established in 1965, when the Bureau of Health and Hospitals of the former National Catholic Welfare Conference formed the Catholic chaplains' association. By 1970, the NACC had become a recognized chaplain-certifying-and-training organization. In 1973, NACC also began to admit sisters, brothers, and lay persons as certified members of the NACC, calling them pastoral associates. NACC describes itself as "a professional association for certified chaplains and clinical pastoral educators who participate in the healing mission of Jesus Christ. We provide standards, certification, education, advocacy and professional development for our members in service to the Church and society."[3]

The National Association of Jewish Chaplains (NAJC) seeks to "enhance the kedusha of Jewish Chaplains in order that they may provide quality Jewish, religious, and spiritual care." NAJC describes itself further as

> a professional organization for Rabbis, Cantors, and other Jewish professionals functioning as Jewish Chaplains in hospitals, nursing homes and geriatric centers, hospice, psychiatric facilities, correctional centers, and the military. In addition to offering collegial support to and professional certification of Jewish Chaplains, NAJC provides conferences and ongoing resources to its members to foster services to and resources for the Jewish and general community on issues of pastoral and spiritual care based on Jewish traditions and values.[4]

NAJC puts on an annual conference and publishes a journal and a quarterly newsletter.

Each of these organizations set the standards for certification for members. These standards are generally similar across organizations, and include a master's degree in theology, divinity, religious studies, or pastoral ministry granted by an accredited academic institution, and four units of Clinical Pastoral Education (CPE) (1,625 hours of clinical supervision counseling medically ill persons called a "residency") from an accredited CPE center. APC also requires one year of full-time chaplaincy experience after residency. In addition, a letter of endorsement is required from the chaplain's denomination and successful passing of both a written and an oral board exam is required to become a Board Certified Chaplain (BCC). Furthermore, APC and NACC require at least fifty hours of continuing education (CE) a year through participation in a broad range of educational experiences, and APC requires that ten of these hours must be approved as Continuing Chaplain Education (CCE) units. APC also has an associate chaplain category that requires one (instead of 4 units) of CPE and requires fewer CE units per year to maintain certification. NAJC also requires ongoing continuing education to maintain certification. Although the proportion of chaplains in the United States who are board certified (BCC) is unknown, many hospitals are now seeking chaplains with these credentials.

The Association for Clinical Pastoral Education (ACPE) is the organization that sets the standards for clinical pastoral education, accredits CPE centers and programs, and certifies supervisors in CPE.[5] ACPE was established in 1967 with the merging of the Institute of Pastoral Care, the Council for Clinical Training, the Association of Clinical Pastoral Educators, and the certification and accreditation functions of the Lutheran Council. CPE had its origins in the 1920s as a form of theological education that took place in both academic classrooms and clinical settings. Pastoral care departments at large hospitals or medical centers today often include ACPE-certified programs for the training of chaplains.

What Chaplains Do

Board-certified chaplains are trained to comprehensively assess the spiritual needs of patients and to then address those needs. Chaplains are trained to do this for patients from a wide range of religious traditions and for those with no religious tradition. Besides Protestant, Catholic, and Jewish chaplains, there are also Buddhist, Hindu, and Muslim chaplains. Although associated with a specific religious tradition, chaplains are ecumenically trained and able to provide spiritual and religious support to patients and families of all faiths. In the hospital setting, chaplains are the true spiritual care specialists, and are the only professionals within the health care field who are specifically trained to meet spiritual needs that arise during medical or psychiatric illness. Chaplains may either be generalists or specialize in pre- or postsurgical care, adult care, geriatrics, pediatrics, oncology, or the care of the dying (hospice).

Chaplains hold chapel services and administer the sacraments at the bedside, as well as pray with and counsel patients, family members, and hospital staff. Chaplains also serve on ethics committees and institutional review boards, participate in discharge planning, and liaison with community clergy. In some hospitals (ideally), chaplains are an integral part of the multidisciplinary health care team, participating in bedside hospital rounds on patients and attending multidisciplinary team meetings. Chaplains are often involved in controversial ethical questions, such as removing ventilator support or feeding tubes, other conflicts related to end-of-life decisions, patient refusal of treatment on religious grounds, treatment of the developmentally delayed, and so on, and chaplains receive special training to handle such issues. Chaplains serve a unique role on ethics committees in identifying and clarifying a patient's spiritual and moral perspectives, and in determining how these might impact decision making.[6] Chaplains are especially helpful to patients, families and staff during times of crisis such as might occur in intensive care units, emergency rooms, and hospice settings.

What chaplains spend their time doing, however, is dependent on how many chaplains the hospital has on staff. Hospitals vary tremendously on the number of chaplains they hire, how they hire them, and the qualifications of persons they call chaplains. Hospitals may have as many as one chaplain per one hundred beds, one chaplain per five hundred beds, or no chaplains at all. Chaplains may be full time (with benefits), part time (limited benefits), or contracted (paid by the hour, no benefits). Chaplains may or may not be board certified, although some hospitals are requiring this credentialing. When the needs of a hospital are greater than the chaplain can provide, he or she may recruit clergy from the community to help out. Many different models exist. Some hospitals have volunteer chaplain programs and visiting clergy programs (involving community clergy or trained volunteers), which are usually coordinated by the hospital's department of pastoral care and directed by a full-time chaplain. Hospitals may have a separate department of pastoral care, or pastoral care may be part of the department of social services.

Nursing homes typically do not have chaplains unless a nursing home is religiously affiliated, in which case it may or may not have a chaplain on staff. Outpatient medical and psychiatric clinics also do not typically have chaplains. Of course, people confined to home who receive home health services seldom have the option of seeing a chaplain, and must depend on their community clergy. Chaplains are not the same as community clergy. Community clergy may have some training in addressing the needs of sick people, but it is nowhere near the amount or depth that chaplains receive. Most patients, family members, and hospital staff cannot get from their community clergy what they can obtain from a chaplain. The chaplain works in the health care setting, understands the psychological and social consequences of illness, and knows how to "walk alongside" those who are struggling with illness and with those who are caring for them. The chaplain knows the doctors and nurses and the hospital procedures and understands the ethics of health care. Chaplains are members of the hospital staff and may attend multidisciplinary team meetings, and so will have access to medical, nursing, and social information relevant to patient care. Community clergy do not have such connections or knowledge, and so simply cannot be as helpful to patients and family as chaplains can.

Chaplain Assessment

There are no standard chaplain assessment tools used by all chaplains. Instead, each pastoral care department determines what works best in its particular setting, tailored to individual patients. It is the patient's needs and beliefs that guide the evaluation. Nevertheless, there is general agreement on what needs to be included in a chaplain's spiritual assessment, and this follows closely the requirements of the Joint Commission for Accreditation of Hospital Organizations.[7] Thus, depending on what the screening spiritual history by the HP reveals, the chaplain will conduct a more comprehensive assessment that will explore further the patient's beliefs and spiritual needs, while following the patient's lead in areas covered. These evaluations are always *patient centered*.

Unfortunately, most chaplains are in work situations where they simply do not have the time to see every patient and family member, as well as address the needs of hospital staff and fulfill their other hospital-related responsibilities. The result is that only one in five hospitalized patients sees a chaplain,[8] and even fewer family members have an opportunity to talk with chaplains. For this reason, it is important to prioritize the tasks for which chaplains are responsible. Screening every single patient for spiritual needs is not something that most chaplains need to do or can do (except in military or veterans administration hospital settings). Not all patients will have spiritual needs, want to talk about them with someone, or desire to see a chaplain.

For these reasons, it makes more sense for non-chaplain HPs to screen patients in order to acquire this information, and then refer patients who have spiritual needs to the chaplain. This way, the HP can also explain to the patient what a chaplain actually does (most patients have no idea what chaplains do or their qualifications) and encourage the patient to see the chaplain if spiritual needs are present and are affecting the patient's coping and/or medical decisions.

A number of specific models of pastoral care in hospital settings have been developed by chaplains such as Gary Fitchett[9] at Rush-Presbyterian Hospital in Chicago and Arthur Lucas[10] at Barnes-Jewish Hospital in St. Louis, which are sometimes used as a basis for spiritual assessment and intervention. Chaplain Gary Berg at the Veterans Administration Medical Center in White Cloud, Minnesota, has also developed a computerized spiritual assessment tool.[11] This tool includes a "spiritual injury" scale that asks patients if they never, sometimes, often, or very often experienced spiritual injuries. These include guilt, shame, rage, grief, unfair treatment by God or life, and other injuries to their religious worldview. The reader should turn to these sources for more information.

Chaplain Interventions

After assessment, the chaplain will develop a spiritual care plan tailored to the patient's specific needs. In some circumstances, the chaplain will not even talk about God or religious topics, but will instead use whatever language the patient uses to delve into things that are important to the patient (concerns about loved ones, meaning and purpose, physical pain and suffering, fears about death or dying, etc.). The chaplain may not even pray with the patient unless this is something the patient wants. Before any spiritual intervention, the chaplain will seek permission from the patient. The chaplain may or may not contact the patient's clergy, depending on the patient's particular needs and preferences. As with assessment, chaplain interventions are always *patient centered*. The chaplain will tailor assessments and interventions to the patient's faith tradition, whatever that may be, and will never evangelize patients or coerce patients to believe or practice in a certain way. According to the chaplain code of ethics, the chaplain absolutely respects the patient's freedom of choice and always serves as the advocate of the patient in health care–related matters.[12]

Chaplains are also available to meet the emotional and spiritual needs of hospital staff. This is especially true for nurses and other HPs working on units within the hospital, and is becoming increasingly true for physicians who are experiencing high job stress. One study found that 73 percent of intensive care physicians and nurses indicated that providing comfort for staff is an important role of the chaplain, and many also felt that chaplains should be available to help staff with personal problems as well.[13] The chaplain makes every effort to get to know hospital staff and develop relationships with them. This serves many purposes. First, HPs get to know chaplains and learn what they do (like patients, most HPs don't know about the training of chaplains and the areas in which they can be helpful). Second, from the chaplain's perspective, developing a personal relationship with the HPs will increase patient referrals. Third, getting to know the

HPs will increase the likelihood that chaplains will be included as part of the multidisciplinary team (if this is not already occurring). HPs are always faced with difficult ethical decisions, problem patients, or patients with specific spiritual needs. Having a good relationship with the chaplain will enable the HP to readily call on that chaplain for help. HPs may find that the chaplain can assist them with their own issues related to caring for patients and dealing with colleagues. The chaplain is often seen as someone who can be trusted to keep things confidential, which may not be the case when HPs talk to other colleagues.[14]

Special Needs of Isolation

Patients in acute inpatient settings, long-term care settings, and many of those who are homebound are isolated from their religious communities. Like a soldier in a foreign country or an incarcerated prisoner, these patients have no one in the place where they are confined, other than the chaplain, who is trained to meet their spiritual needs. Patients cannot expect the leaders of their faith communities to visit them in these settings, perform religious rituals, pray, or provide in-depth spiritual counsel related to the health problems they are having.

First, most community clergy simply don't have time to do this, especially if they have large or aging congregations. As much of a problem as this is in acute hospital settings, the situation is even more dire in long-term care settings such as nursing homes. Second, community clergy (and members of the congregation who may be sent in their place) are often not trained to address psychological, social, and spiritual issues related to medical or psychiatric illness. Psychological needs related to illness such as meaning, hope, and purpose, which directly affect rehabilitation and medical outcomes, are closely related to spiritual needs and are often met as spiritual needs are addressed. The same applies to social needs related to illness (being a burden on others, having to live separated from loved ones, and ultimately having to leave loved ones at death). The chaplain is trained to address these complex psychological and social needs that often overlap with spiritual needs. Third, many patients do not have community clergy. At least one-quarter of Americans are "unchurched" (have not attended a religious service in past six months) and will therefore not have clergy to meet their spiritual needs when they are hospitalized.[15]

The same applies to hospital staff, who may be experiencing psychological, social, and spiritual needs as a result of working with sick patients day in and day out, many of whom are suffering and may die in the hospital under their care. Hospital staff need experts with training on the spiritual and psychological needs of those caring for patients with physical or psychiatric illness, chronic disability, and the dying, experts who are readily available to help hospital staff deal with the powerful issues that their jobs force them to confront. Even if staff have their own community clergy, those clergy will not have the kind of training or work as closely with hospital staff or patients as do chaplains.

Thus, hospitals and health systems are obligated to hire chaplains to meet the psychological, social, and spiritual needs of patients, families, and hospital staff, who cannot get these needs met in the same way elsewhere. Chaplains serve the special needs of patients, families, and staff who are isolated because of their confinement or type of work. The medical knowledge, training in medical and psychiatric counseling, and connection with other members of the health care team uniquely qualify chaplains to serve the emotional, social, and spiritual needs of these people.

Chaplains also have special training that prepares them to serve many other functions in the hospital, from serving on ethics committees and institutional review boards to mobilizing assistance from the patient's faith community after discharge. Again, unless they have the extensive training that a chaplain has, most clergy working outside of the health care system simply cannot do this.

PASTORAL COUNSELORS

While chaplains and community clergy do plenty of counseling, the term "pastoral counselor" usually refers to a specific kind of mental health professional. Pastoral counselors are particularly important for meeting the spiritual and psychological needs of patients in situations where chaplains are not available, such as in the outpatient setting. The American Association of Pastoral Counselors (AAPC) is the national membership organization that sets standards and certifies pastoral counselors. AAPC describes pastoral counseling as

> a unique form of psychotherapy which uses spiritual resources as well as psychological understanding for healing and growth. Pastoral counselors are certified mental health professionals who have had in-depth religious and/or theological training. . . . Pastoral counseling moves beyond the support or encouragement a religious community can offer, by providing psychologically sound therapy that weaves in the religious and spiritual dimension.[16]

Founded in 1963, AAPC has a membership that now exceeds three thousand and provides nearly three million hours of counseling per year in institutional and private settings. The qualifications needed for certification include four years of college, three years of divinity school or seminary, and a master's or doctoral degree in counseling or psychology. This includes at least

1,375 hours of supervised clinical experience involving individual, group, marital and family therapy, and 250 hours of direct approved supervision working in both acute and long-term care settings. Pastoral counselors can be especially useful in private medical, surgical, and psychiatric outpatient clinics where chaplains are not available and complex psychological and spiritual issues often come up. As health care moves more and more into the outpatient setting, the role of pastoral counselors will become increasingly important. The AAPC Web site provides the ability to search for a local pastoral counselor anywhere in the United States.[17]

COMMUNITY CLERGY

Community clergy, while not as extensively trained on how to address health-related spiritual needs and not positioned within the health care system in a way that connects them to patients' health care providers (as are chaplains), nevertheless play an important role in helping to meet the patient's spiritual needs both in the hospital and after the patient is discharged back into the community. Depending on the denomination of the religious congregation, its size, and age composition, clergy may be expected to visit members of the congregation when they are in the hospital. These visits, or visits by clergy "extenders" (volunteers from within the faith community), are important for helping patients feel connected to and cared for by their religious communities.

Many community clergy also have specific training in clinical pastoral education (CPE), which may be required for ordination by their denomination (1 unit of CPE), or they may acquire such training from hospital chaplains whom they assist and even take calls for. Community clergy often make extraordinary efforts to visit sick members of their congregation and provide those members with support, encouragement, and spiritual counsel, both in and outside the hospital.

Finally, visits by clergy may be an important time when HPs can talk with them (with patient consent) about patients' spiritual needs identified during hospitalization that will need follow-up. After discharge, patients' clergy and faith community will often be the only sources of spiritual care and practical assistance that are available to them. Thus, good communication between HPs, hospital chaplains, and clergy is essential so that continuity of spiritual care can be maintained from hospital to community.

SUMMARY AND CONCLUSIONS

While HPs without religious training serve key roles in identifying spiritual issues related to health care and determining if patients have specific spiritual needs, they are usually not able to address those needs. Chaplains, pastoral counselors, and community clergy each serve unique and different roles in helping patients who are acutely hospitalized, in nursing homes, or in outpatient settings. Chaplains have special expertise in addressing the spiritual, psychological, and social needs of hospitalized patients, and serve many other crucial functions that enable hospitals to operate efficiently and ethically. Pastoral counselors are trained to address the psychological and social needs of medical and psychiatric patients in outpatient settings where chaplains are not available. Community clergy are responsible for following up on spiritual needs identified during hospitalization and mobilizing members of the faith community to meet the practical needs of patients after discharge in terms of psychological, social, and spiritual support. It is essential that HPs understand what chaplains, pastoral counselors, and community clergy can do, the kind of training they receive, and how they approach patients in clinical settings, so that HPs can appropriately refer patients and inform patients what these spiritual care specialists have to offer.

CHAPTER 8

SPIRITUALITY IN NURSING CARE

In this chapter, I address spirituality within nursing but, given the limited space, this is done in only the most superficial and general manner. For readers who want more in-depth information on this very large topic, there are other texts authored by nurse professionals that deal with the subject matter much more comprehensively (especially with regard to applications in clinical practice).[1]

The profession of nursing emerged out of religious orders that provided care to the sick. Until the past hundred years or so, almost all nursing care in the Western world was done by women religious (i.e., deaconesses from the Protestant tradition or sisters from the Catholic tradition). This was true in the United States as well as in Europe. The first organized group of nurses in the United States was the Sisters of Charity in Emmitsburg, Maryland, established in 1803. Until the 1960s, many nurses lived in dormitories next to the hospital in which they worked, and often were unmarried (following the same model as Catholic sisters). Only in recent times has nursing become "evidence based" and departed from its religious origins. Over the past thirty years, U.S. nursing has become more and more secularized, seldom emphasizing the spiritual needs of patients either in training or in practice. By the time I went to nursing school in the late 1970s, spirituality had been almost completely expunged from the curriculum. If a nurse was caught praying with a patient or discussing spiritual issues, it could mean reprimand or dismissal.

Despite the purging of spirituality from nurses' training during the 1970s and 1980s, even during these years, there were nurse leaders who continued to emphasize the importance of spirituality in nursing care. In *Spiritual Dimensions of Nursing Practice*, published in 1989 by Saunders, Verna Benner Carson describes the role of the nurses in identifying and addressing the spiritual needs of patients.[2] Even before that, in 1981, Margaret Colliton wrote a chapter titled "Spiritual Dimension of Nursing" in the fourth edition of *Clinical Nursing*, published by Macmillan,[3] and in 1975, Jean Stallwood and Ruth Stall wrote a chapter by the same title in the third edition of the text.[4] So, within clinical nursing, spirituality has always been recognized at some level.

Although the pendulum has begun to swing back in recent years, today a deep divide remains between nursing care and spiritual care. The requirement by JCAHO that a spiritual history be done on every patient admitted to the hospital, nursing home, or seen by a home health agency has encouraged nurses to once again address these issues. Although there is no research that documents to what extent spiritual histories are actually being taken by nurses in U.S. hospitals, it is my impression that this is an area being only superficially addressed. Yes, many nurses may determine the religious denomination of the patient and whether the patient wants to see a chaplain or not, but that is *not* a spiritual history—or anything close to what is required by JCAHO. Systematic research is desperately needed to understand what is being done, what is not done, and why.

NURSING RESEARCH

At least preliminary research on nurses addressing spiritual issues in clinical care does exist, however, and I will review some of that research now.

Identifying Spiritual Needs. JCAHO began discussing the possibility of including a spiritual care criterion in 1998, and in the year 2000, the spiritual history requirement became official.[5] Despite this criterion, to my knowledge, no systematic research has yet examined the proportion of hospital nurses in the United States who regularly do a spiritual history of the quality and depth recommended by JCAHO. According to some nursing experts, registered nurses infrequently conduct spiritual assessments or identify spiritual needs.[6]

Providing Spiritual Care. With regard to providing spiritual *care*, 71 percent of 299 nurses at a large university hospital in the southwestern United States reported that they had at some time offered, suggested, or provided prayer to patients.[7] More than a quarter (29%) indicated that they had offered spiritual counseling. Nearly all nurses (96–98%) indicated that they would "offer, suggest or provide" spiritual help if the patient explicitly requested spiritual support or were about to die. In this study, however, a broad definition of spirituality was used that included holding a patient's hand, listening, or use of laughter. To my knowledge, this is the only study of U.S. hospital nurses on spiritual care behaviors. The only other nursing study that I could find, now almost fifteen years old, found that 100 percent of British nurses indicated that patients had spiritual needs, but 67 percent said that patients' spiritual needs were either poorly met or not met at all; 60 percent of nurses expressed a desire to have more education on spiritual care.[8]

More is known about the spiritual care behaviors of nurse practitioners (NPs) in the U.S. than is known for hospital nurses. A 2001 survey of 102 NPs found that 57 percent rarely or never provided spiritual care, which they explained as due to lack of formal education related to spiritual care. When spiritual care was provided, it involved primarily praying privately for patients or referring them to a member of the clergy.[9] Most recently, a 2006 survey of sixty-five nurse practitioners in the Bible Belt (North Carolina) found that 73 percent did not routinely provide spiritual care to patients, 61 percent only rarely or occasionally "talked with my patient about a spiritual and/or religious topic," and 92 percent only rarely or occasionally prayed with a patient.[10] Likewise, 47 percent only rarely or occasionally referred patients to a religious leader and 71 percent only rarely or occasionally referred patients to hospital chaplains. If this is the case in the most religious area of the country, it is likely that NPs do even less elsewhere.

Nursing Education. In a study of 176 nurses in 1990, researchers report that while 97 percent believed that whole person nursing care involved spiritual care, nearly two-thirds (65.9%) said they were not adequately prepared to provide spiritual care.[11] In a 1996 study of mental health nurses, 76 percent reported that they had received no education on spirituality in their nursing program.[12] More recent articles continue to report that nursing education is woefully inadequate in preparing nurses to address the spiritual needs of patients, and many nurses feel unprepared to do this.[13]

A recent study, though, suggests that things may be improving. Lemmer surveyed 132 of 250 randomly selected baccalaureate nursing programs in the United States.[14] The focus was on whether or not these programs included spirituality in their curricula. The results of this study, however, likely present a "best-case scenario," since 39 percent of the programs that responded to the survey were sponsored by religious organizations, and nursing schools that did not address spirituality may have been less likely to return the questionnaire. In any case, 97 percent of programs said they included spirituality in the curriculum and 71 percent said they included the spiritual dimension in their programs' philosophy. On a scale of 1 (strongly disagree) to 5 (strongly agree), the statement "Spiritual care is a significant part of nursing care" received an average rating of 4.2. With regard to content, assessment of spiritual needs received an average rating of 2.9 (where 1 = not taught at all; 2 = covered briefly; 3 = covered to a moderate degree; 4 = covered in depth). With regard to training in use of a formal spiritual assessment tool, the average rating was 1.5.

Two-thirds (65%) of programs said they addressed spiritual factors during the first two years, and 82 percent said they integrated spiritual care concepts throughout the nursing curricula (devoting an average of 7 hours to the topic). However, there was widespread disagreement on the definition of spirituality (87%) and on the definition of spiritual nursing care (94%).

In Canada, the situation appears to be similarly grave. In a 2003 survey of twenty-nine Canadian university schools of nursing (undergraduate curricula), eighteen schools responded.[15] The findings were that spirituality was rarely defined or included in curricular objectives.

Reasons for Neglect. There are probably many reasons why nurses are not assessing or addressing spiritual issues more regularly. Unfortunately, very little is known about the barriers that are responsible for this, although they are probably similar to those reported by physicians. I could find only one systematic study that addressed this issue for nurses. In this 1987 study, three-quarters (76%) of oncology nurses indicated that lack of time was a factor preventing their routinely conducting a spiritual assessment.[16] Based on reports by nurses from studies cited above, lack of emphasis during nurses' training is another important reason why many nurses who trained in the 1970s, 1980s, and 1990s do not routinely ask about spiritual issues.

WHAT SHOULD NURSES DO?

Here are some practical suggestions on what nurses can do to integrate spirituality into nursing care. As I indicated earlier, there are more developed texts written by nursing leaders that address spiritual distress as a nursing diagnosis, discuss how to develop a nursing spiritual care plan, and describe how to provide compassionate, sensitive moral and ethical care to patients. Here is what I recommend (much of which is repetitive from other sections of this book).

Take a Spiritual History. During every new patient evaluation, whether that involves admission to the hospital for a medical or psychiatric admission, admission to a nursing home or rehabilitation setting, or when seeing a homebound patient as part of home health care, always take a spiritual history (unless already performed and documented by a physician or chaplain). This is the one aspect of integrating spirituality into patient care that cannot be avoided. It is required by JCAHO, and it opens up a dialogue with the patient about spiritual issues if they are important to the patient. Taking the spiritual history will communicate to the patient that this is a topic that he or she can talk about with the nurse. Keep the spiritual history brief and general, and remember that this is mainly about *information gathering*, not about intervention. Any of the spiritual histories recommended in this book will serve the purpose. The aim is to collect information about the patient's spiritual beliefs that could be relevant to the medical or nursing care of the patient. Next, document this information in the medical record in a designated area of the chart.

Support the Beliefs of the Patient. Support and show respect for the religious beliefs of the patient. Recognize that those beliefs often serve a purpose, and the ability of the patient to cope may depend on them. If the nurse feels the religious beliefs of the patient are unhealthy or conflicting with care, then the nurse should talk with the chaplain and discuss the possibility of involving the patient's clergy. The nurse should not attempt to change or challenge those religious beliefs. Again, the chaplain will be an invaluable resources in ambiguous cases.

Pray with Patient. If the patient desires and requests it (and the nurse is open to doing it), then I think prayer with patients is permissible. However, the nurse should follow the suggestions in earlier chapters on how to go about this and what conditions should be present to reduce the possibility of coercion.

Provide Spiritual Care. By this, I mean that whatever you do with, to, or for the patient, do it in a kind, gentle, sensitive, and compassionate manner. Treat every patient as the image of God that he or she is. In the Christian tradition, the one that I am most familiar with, Jesus washed his disciples' feet at the Last Supper. He did this carefully and lovingly, to show them the importance of serving each other. So also, we should serve patients with kindness and loving care, showing respect for the person and his or her uniqueness. By uniqueness, I mean that every patient is different from every other patient, and will have different needs, hopes, and dreams. Treating each patient as special, as important, as *relevant*—this is perhaps the heart of spiritual care. No mention of God or Jesus or Moses or Muhammad or Buddha is necessary, unless that is what the patient wants to talk about. Granted, this is a pretty broad definition of spiritual care (especially given my comments in chapter 1 about definitions), but I'm not sure if nurses are really qualified to go much beyond this. Of course, opinions will vary, and I encourage the reader to turn to nursing texts on spiritual care.

Refer to Pastoral Care. If the patient will allow it, the nurse should refer any spiritual needs that come up during the spiritual history to pastoral care professionals. They are the ones trained to provide spiritual care in the formal sense, and should be deferred to in all cases if available. Make full use of the training, experience, and skills of chaplains. Nurses should try to get to know the hospital chaplains so that if emotional or spiritual issues come up in the course of their work (patient related or personal), they will feel comfortable talking about them with the chaplain.

Nurses and Chaplains Are Natural Allies and Should Not Be Competing to Meet the Spiritual Needs of Patients. Nurses depend on chaplains to take care of spiritual needs that they don't have the time or training to address, and chaplains depend on nurses for many of their referrals. We found that 49 percent of physicians made no referrals for chaplain services and only 5 percent made ten or more referrals during the previous six months, compared to only 14 percent of nurses making no referrals and 47 percent making ten or more.[17] Similarly, a more recent survey of nurses, social workers, and physicians at Memorial Sloan Kettering Cancer Center in New York City found that 82 percent of chaplain referrals were made by nurses, 12 percent by social workers, and 4 percent by physicians.[18]

SUMMARY AND CONCLUSIONS

No health care professional spends more time with the patient than the nurse, and the nurse spends time with *every* patient. Until recently, nursing care was the province and domain of women religious. Almost everything that a nurse does with, to, or for the patient can be carried out in a spiritual manner; however, some of what the nurse does must have an explicit spiritual component. This involves taking a spiritual history, particularly if the physician or chaplain has not already done so and documented it (and this will not have been done in most cases). It also involves support-ing the beliefs of the patient, praying with patients on occasion if requested, and referring to pastoral care any spiritual needs that require addressing. Nurses should receive training during nurs-ing school so that they will feel comfortable communicating with patients about spiritual issues and learn what to do when spiritual needs come up. That training should be based on state-of-the-art research done by nurses and integrated throughout the nursing curriculum in an explicit way.

CHAPTER 9

SPIRITUALITY IN SOCIAL WORK

Because spiritual and religious issues bear on the patient's psychological state and social environment, social workers may be called upon to identify the religious or spiritual resources of patients and ensure that spiritual needs are addressed during transitions from hospital to community or community to hospital. There are now a number of special social work interest groups and independent associations that focus on this topic, including the North American Association of Christians in Social Work,[1] Society for Spirituality and Social Work,[2] Canadian Society for Spirituality and Social Work,[3] and Center for Spirituality and Integral Social Work at The Catholic University of America.[4] There is even a *Journal of Religion & Spirituality in Social Work* that publishes research and discussions on spiritual issues in social work. Furthermore, at least two edited books and one authored book have been published by social workers on the topic.[5] Despite the growing interest, however, there is almost no content on addressing spiritual issues in most courses required to obtain a master's degree in social work.[6]

SOCIAL WORK RESEARCH

Systematic research provides information on the attitudes and activities of social workers related to assessing and addressing spiritual needs. A survey of 221 social workers in the southeastern United States revealed that religious-based interventions were judged appropriate by more than 50 percent of respondents and utilized by that percentage as well. High personal spirituality predicted positive attitudes and utilization.[7] A survey of 299 gerontological social workers found that most respondents supported the inclusion of religion and spirituality in education and practice as part of diversity and holistic assessment.[8] However, nearly 70 percent reported little or no preparation on spiritual issues during their social work education and less than 25 percent said they were satisfied by the preparation they received.

Sheridan surveyed a random sample of 204 licensed social workers, finding that there was considerable focus on religion and spirituality in both social work assessments and interventions.[9] More then two-thirds of the sample reported they had utilized one of fourteen different spiritually derived techniques with clients. Again, however, practitioners' own personal beliefs and level of participation in religious or spiritual services predicted their use of spiritual techniques. Hodge describes an instrument called the "spiritual lifemap" that can be used in spiritual assessments by social workers. He indicates that it facilitates the transition from taking a spiritual history to planning interventions, and his article provides several cases to illustrate the instrument's use.[10]

Thus, there is considerable attention being paid by many social workers to spiritual issues, despite the fact that training on why, how, and when to assess and address spiritual issues has often been absent in social work education. Instead, as with physicians and nurses, it is the personal religiousness or spirituality of the practitioner that determines whether this topic is addressed. Again, HP activities in this area should be driven by training, importance of the subject to patients, and relationship to health and support, not by the personal beliefs of the practitioner.

WHAT SHOULD SOCIAL WORKERS DO?

The ultimate goal of social workers is to improve people's lives by providing counseling, advice, and direction, and by connecting them with resources. Medical social workers work with patients and families in planning discharge from the hospital back into the community, into either a safe independent living situation or a long-term care or rehabilitation setting . The medical social worker is the primary liaison person between the hospital and the community. The community social worker plays a similar role, although the focus can sometimes be in the other direction—helping people move from the community into a hospital or long-term care setting. Community social workers often see individuals struggling with some kind of social problem, such as inadequate housing, unemployment, poverty, a serious illness (physical and mental), a disability, or substance abuse. They also work with families that have serious domestic conflicts, involving children or adults who are being abused in some way.

Thus, social workers seek out resources within the community to help support people and enable them either to live independently in the community or to find another living situation that is safe and secure. They also do a lot of individual and family counseling, often when people are at a low point in their lives. The social worker, then, is ideally positioned to screen for and address spiritual issues that come up when discharging patients from the hospital or when transitioning them from the community into another community setting or institution. These kinds of transitions are always stressful, and religious faith can play a big role in helping people to cope with such changes and in providing them with the community support that can help make transitions successful.

The medical social worker should be familiar with the patient's religious background and experiences. This information can be gathered from the spiritual history taken by the physician, nurse, or chaplain, and can be supplemented with information gathered directly from the patient. Of course, if no spiritual history has yet been done and documented, then the social worker should be the person who does it. A much abbreviated spiritual history may also be necessary at the time of discharge (i.e., a question such as, "Were your spiritual needs met to your satisfaction during your hospital stay; are there still some issues that you need some help with?"). With this information, the social worker can determine if there are any unaddressed spiritual needs that are still present at the time of discharge, and can help to develop a plan to meet those needs in the community after discharge.

The social worker should work closely with the chaplain to develop the discharge spiritual care plan, and depending on who has the available time, either the social worker or chaplain would then implement the plan by contacting the patient's community clergy (after obtaining explicit permission from the patient and documenting this). The discharge spiritual care plan might also include arranging for meals to be brought to the patient by members of the faith community, or perhaps arranging for faith community volunteers to help prepare the patient's home to ensure that the environment is safe (rails built on steps, commode raised, seats and rails put in shower, etc.). This might involve members of the faith community working together with an occupational therapist from the hospital.

If there are spiritual needs that remain unmet, for either the patient or the family, then the medical social worker could make arrangements for counseling and support by the patient's clergy or other trained individual within or outside the faith community. Spiritual needs might involve unresolved grief over loss of independence or loss of loved ones, spiritual struggles related to anger at God for unanswered prayers, fears about what will happen after death, or desire for guidance on how to deepen one's religious faith or relationship with God. For homebound patients or patients moving into a nursing home, the spiritual care plan may involve arranging for someone from the faith community to visit the patient, pray with or read religious scriptures to the patient, administer religious sacraments such as the Holy Eucharist, or help the patient perform some other religious ritual that is important to him or her (perhaps arrange transportation to attend worship services, obtain access to foods so that a kosher diet can be followed, etc.).

Community social workers may have many similar roles, although often they will not have a chaplain readily available to consult. Instead, the social worker may want to develop a relationship with a chaplain or trained pastoral counselor in the community who can help develop a plan to meet the patient's spiritual needs either in the community or in a new institutional setting. If the patient is from a religious or spiritual faith tradition that is not familiar to the social worker or if pastoral care specialists are not available, then direct contact with the patient's clergy (after permission has been obtained and documented) may be necessary to develop this plan.

Often religious faith is very important and has been a source of strength for many years for people who are having social problems. Helping to provide the spiritual resources necessary for these people to fully mobilize their faith during times of need can be a powerful way to facilitate adaptation during crisis. However, as emphasized earlier in this book, spiritual assessment and interventions should always be patient centered, and there is no room for coercion that interferes with the patient's free and independent choice—a choice that may or *may not* involve spirituality or religion. If a patient is not religious or spiritual, as indicated earlier, special care must be taken to avoid coercion or inducing guilt over such matters. This is particularly true since a social worker may be acting as an agent of the state or hospital system.

SUMMARY AND CONCLUSIONS

Medical and community social workers help patients and families transition from one living situation to another, easing such transitions by providing counsel and identifying resources. Relevant to such transitions are the religious/spiritual beliefs of patients and families and the faith communities to which they belong. As part of holistic, patient-centered care, there is growing interest among social workers to identify the spiritual needs of patients and families and to ensure that those spiritual needs are met during such transitions. Medical social workers are ideally positioned to ensure that spiritual needs identified during hospitalization continue to be addressed as patients are discharged back into the community. This is often done by working closely with the chaplain to locate resources either within or outside of the patient's religious community to meet those needs, depending on the patient's choice. Community social workers play a similar but broader role that involves identifying spiritual needs and identifying spiritual resources in an environment where pastoral care specialists may not be readily available.

In hospital settings, the medical social worker should not duplicate the work of physicians, nurses, or chaplains in identifying spiritual needs, although he or she may have to conduct and document a spiritual history if it has not already been done, and may need to follow up briefly at the time of discharge to ensure that spiritual needs were met during hospitalization. Because most social workers are not trained to address spiritual issues, however, any in-depth spiritual counseling should be left to pastoral care specialists whenever this option is available.

CHAPTER 10

SPIRITUALITY IN REHABILITATION

Physical and occupational therapists treat patients who are recovering from accidents, injuries, and acute medical or surgical illnesses. They also work with those who have chronic illness who are seeking to regain or maximize their independence and functioning. Many of these patients may rely on religious or spiritual beliefs to cope with the stresses involved in recovery, and there is evidence that religious faith may be a key factor in helping patients to stay motivated and not give up. Not surprisingly, then, many physical and occupational therapists are looking for a role in assessing and addressing the spiritual needs of their patients.

There now exist several Christian and non-Christian associations that focus on these issues. Among the Christian associations are the Christian Physical Therapists International[1] and International Occupational Therapists for Christ.[2] There are also multicultural networking groups designated within the American Occupational Therapy

Association (AOTA) that include the Association of Asian/Pacific Occupational Therapists in America, the Network for Native American Practitioners, and the Orthodox Jewish Occupational Therapy Caucus.[3] Although I could not locate other religious PT or OT groups that address the spiritual needs of patients and therapists, it is likely that others exist.

To get a sense of what the Christian organizations do, an examination of their Web sites reveals the following. Christian Physical Therapists International seeks to "encourage, support and build you spiritually and professionally; to help you have an impact on your profession through your faith; and to help you meet your colleagues' and clients' spiritual needs, too."[4] The International Occupational Therapists for Christ has similar aims that include "glorifying God through the excellent and Godly practice of our profession. The organization promotes the knowledgeable integration of factors of spirituality into a comprehensive approach to health, the evidence based best practice of occupational therapy, the provision of service to underserved populations locally and internationally and supports members' faith in their practice of Christian occupational therapy."

The AOTA networking groups each have a specific mission related to cultural or spiritual issues. The Association of Asian/ Pacific Occupational Therapists in America states that its mission is to "create a means for the occupational therapy practitioners who are committed to supporting Asian/Pacific practitioners and advancing a greater understanding of Asian/Pacific cultural issues affecting occupational therapy practice." The Network for Native American Practitioners (NNAP) says it seeks to "increase resources for occupational therapists currently working with, or interested in working with, Native Americans. The NNAP promotes the recruitment and retention of Native Americans into the field of occupational therapy and the development of materials to educate the profession and the AOTA membership about Native American issues."

The Orthodox Jewish Occupational Therapy Caucus is more explicit in its dealing with religious issues in seeking to

> provide a forum for personal and professional networking for Jewish Occupational Therapists and OT students, . . . work with our professional organizations to help them meet the religious needs of our members when it comes to arranging and scheduling conferences, seminars and other opportunities for professional growth, . . . provide a forum for our members and other occupational therapists to discuss issues relating to practice of our profession and our religion, [and] . . . assist our members in dealing with conflicts that arise in the areas of Shabbat and Kashrut and similar religious matters.

Thus, each of these groups appears to support the cultural, religious, and spiritual growth of therapists themselves and/or address the spiritual needs of patients as they arise in clinical practice.

REHABILITATION RESEARCH

What do we know from systematic research about the interest in or activity of rehabilitation specialists regarding integrating spirituality into patient care? When patients experience loss of ability to function, PT and OT help them to resume some kind of meaningful daily activity. Because religious or spiritual involvement appears to help patients with medical illness to cope and give life a sense of purpose and meaning, studies have examined the attitudes of physical and occupational therapists toward addressing these issues.

In a survey of 136 physical therapists employed in clinics in Michigan associated with the physical therapy department of

Andrews University, 96 percent agreed that spirituality is an important component of good health, although only 44 percent indicated that they should address spiritual concerns of patients and over 50 percent never discussed issues related to spirituality with patients.[5] Another recent study provides information about the attitudes of physical therapists toward including spirituality in their training. That study sampled 166 faculty from 101 physical therapy education programs in the U.S.[6] Nearly half (49%) indicated their PT programs included spirituality concepts, and 56 percent said they believed spirituality concepts should be included in PT education. The general opinion was that rather than have specific courses on it, spirituality should be integrated throughout the PT curriculum.

With regard to occupational therapy, as early as 1991, the Canadian Association of Occupational Therapy and the Department of National Health and Welfare developed guidelines on addressing spiritual issues in OT, from initial assessment to discharge planning.[7] They based these guidelines on the fact that for many patients, spirituality is their foundation for meaning. In the 1990s, studies both in Canada and the United States indicated that about half of occupational therapists (OT) believed that addressing spirituality in clinical practice was appropriate, whereas others (the majority in the U.S.) felt that this area should be deferred to clergy, since OTs were not adequately trained to address spiritual issues.[8]

More recently, Farrar surveyed 200 Canadian and 210 U.S. occupational therapists, exploring attitudes and practices regarding the spirituality and religious issues in clinical practice.[9] The sample was randomly selected from the membership of the Canadian and American national associations of occupational therapy, with just under 40 percent of subjects responding. Close to 90 percent of respondents indicated that spirituality was an appropriate concern for OTs, with 58 percent already incorporating spirituality into their practice ("spirituality" was broadly defined). About half of therapists (59% in Canada, 46% in the U.S.) assessed the patient's religious affiliation, and most of the time this was used for treatment planning (81% in Canada, 86% in the U.S.) or to mobilize social support from the patient's faith (11% for both Canada and the U.S.).

Thus, the majority of therapists in this study agreed that addressing religious or spiritual issues was appropriate in their line of work. However, OTs were concerned about how to address spiritual issues without imposing their own beliefs, and emphasized the need to keep any activity in this area "client centered." Interestingly, only 6 percent of respondents from both countries indicated that time was a barrier to addressing religious or spiritual issues. In general, attitudes by OTs in the United States were slightly less favorable towards addressing religious or spiritual issues than those in Canada, although differences were not large.

In Farrar's study, therapists provided examples of how they incorporated the patient's spirituality into their work. For religious patients, some OTs used the Bible for page-turning dexterity exercises, whereas others suggested reading religious literature as a stress-reduction method. Another study of 206 OTs found that the three methods used most often in addressing the spiritual needs of patients were: (1) praying for a patient, (2) using spiritual language or concepts, and (3) discussing ways that the patient's religious beliefs were helpful.[10] Rosenfeld emphasized the role of spirituality in "meaning-making," and described eleven prayer activities adapted for the specific needs of disabled patients.[11]

WHAT SHOULD THERAPISTS DO?

In many of the studies cited above, there is no distinction made between "addressing" spiritual issues by therapists and "screening" for spiritual needs by taking a spiritual history. This I think is a crucial distinction. Most PTs or OTs are not trained to "address" spiritual issues or incorporate spiritual treatments into their clinical practice, and so there is valid concern that this activity may not be within their scope of expertise, particularly if there are professional chaplains or pastoral counselors readily available to address these issues. However, taking a spiritual history in order to identify spiritual needs/resources and to better understand the role that these play in the patient's coping with illness, motivation towards recovery, and meaning of life with continuing disability, is quite appropriate and doable for *all* rehabilitation specialists. To my knowledge, however, there are no instruments designed specifically for physical or occupational therapists to guide them on what questions to ask. Until such instruments are developed by therapists tailored to the particular work they do with patients, any of the brief spiritual histories described in this book could be used.

In patients for whom religious or spiritual beliefs are important, supporting those beliefs and perhaps praying with patients if requested (under the circumstances and careful guidelines described earlier) might be some ways that therapists could utilize this information. Even more important, working with pastoral care specialists to address spiritual needs that come up during such discussions is imperative, especially if pastoral care is available and the patient is willing. Even if the patient specifically requests help from the rehabilitation therapist in religious or spiritual matters, it is probably wise for the therapist to seek guidance from a chaplain on how to proceed.

SUMMARY AND CONCLUSIONS

Because religious or spiritual beliefs are important to many patients in rehabilitation settings, and these beliefs are often used to cope with disability and create meaning for illness, this is an area related to the patient's psychological and social functioning that therapists cannot ignore. There are national and international societies of physical and occupational therapists that seek to help members to address religious/spiritual issues in clinical practice and/or to support the religious or spiritual beliefs of members themselves and connect them with others who have similar beliefs. While the vast majority of therapists feel that spirituality is relevant to the care of the patient, only about half say that addressing religious/spiritual issues is appropriate and should be part of their clinical work. My opinion is that the role of rehabilitation therapists in this area lies primarily in taking a spiritual history (or acquiring this information from the medical record), understanding how these factors relate to the rehabilitation of the patient, and supporting the patient's religious or spiritual beliefs that provide comfort and meaning. I would discourage therapists without pastoral care training from addressing the spiritual needs of patients, but instead recommend they work with pastoral care experts, always respecting a patient's choice and never using coercion.

CHAPTER 11

SPIRITUALITY IN
MENTAL HEALTH CARE

T his chapter provides a brief overview of issues related to integrating spirituality into patient care for mental health (MH) professionals. A more thorough treatment of the subject can be found elsewhere in other publications written specifically for psychiatrists,[1] psychologists,[2] and pastoral counselors.[3] These sources also address spirituality from a multireligious perspective, providing perspectives on mental health care from each major religious tradition. This chapter addresses religion and spirituality more generally and largely from a Western religious perspective.

Psychiatrists, psychologists, psychiatric social workers, psychiatric nurses, and mental health counselors provide care to patients with emotional and mental disorders that interfere with their social and occupational functioning and quality of life. For over a century, the divide between health care and religion has been deepest and widest for the mental health specialties. Religion has long been considered neurotic and often inimical to good mental health by MH professionals,[4] and this may have influenced both their own personal beliefs[5] and the value that they attribute to patients' religious or spiritual involvement.[6] Add to this the competition that MH professionals may face from religious professionals, and you have fertile ground for conflict. Competition is evident from the fact that community clergy provide almost as much individual and marital counseling as the entire membership of the American Psychological Association,[7] and often counsel patients with the same range of mental disturbances that MH professionals encounter.[8] Barriers are coming down between these professions, though, and that is encouraging.

RESEARCH ON RELIGION AND MENTAL HEALTH

While there are many deeply religious persons who experience acute or chronic emotional problems, systematic research in samples of medical patients and adults living in the community indicates that those who are more religious tend to have better mental health, not worse. They cope better with illness, experience less depression, and recover more quickly from depression, often experience less anxiety, and have much lower rates of alcohol and drug use.[9] Religious-based psychotherapy has also been shown in randomized clinical trials to speed recovery from depression, bereavement, and generalized anxiety in religious patients, compared to secular therapies or standard care.[10] There is also evidence that persons with severe and persistent mental disorders who are more involved in religious activities cope better with their illnesses and experience less exacerbations requiring acute hospitalization.[11]

Thus, religious beliefs and activities are often valuable resources that help patients cope with difficult situations and may be utilized by MH specialists to help speed recovery or maintain remission from emotional or mental illness. Expert psychiatric care and counseling, combined with the religious resources that patients already have, can often optimize mental health outcomes. Suffering is only increased when one of these approaches is used to the exclusion of the other. For many patients with milder symptoms of depression or anxiety that accompany medical illness or other life stressors, religious belief, practice, and support from the faith community may be enough to help them adapt successfully to difficult circumstances. For patients with more severe or chronic symptoms, those with a personal or family history of emotional problems, and those who are not improving despite religious support, expert psychiatric care is usually needed.

ISSUES IN TREATING PSYCHIATRIC PATIENTS

There are important differences between medical and psychiatric patients that make addressing spiritual issues in clinical practice more difficult. Perhaps the most important difference is the psychological frailty of patients seen by MH specialists and boundary issues that are more important with psychiatric patients than with patients dealing with purely situational or medical problems. For patients with neurotic or psychotic illness, religious beliefs may be distorted and tied to psychiatric symptoms in complex ways.

In the United States, we know that among patients with schizophrenia, 25–39 percent experience religious delusions when psychotic; among patients with bipolar disorder, the rate is 15–22 percent.[12] There is some evidence that religious delusions are associated with more severe symptoms and a worse prognosis over time.[13] This is quite different from nonpsychotic religious beliefs and practices, which, as noted above, usually predict better outcomes and fewer hospitalizations in patients with schizophrenia. Sorting out delusions from non-delusional religious beliefs in these patients, however, is often challenging, and may require the assistance of each patient's clergy.[14] Whether or not religious beliefs are delusional is an important clinical question and may determine whether patients' beliefs are supported or treated with antipsychotic medication.

There is another important difference between medical patients and those seen in MH settings. In psychiatric patients, religion may be intricately tied to the ways they are dealing with the world around them, especially if mental health problems have been present for many years and have roots in childhood (as with chronic depression or personality disorders). Images of God may be distorted by neglectful or abusive parents. Religion may be associated with restrictions and punishments rather than with acceptance, love, mercy, and freedom. Some psychiatric patients are more comfortable in fundamentalist or even cult-like religious settings because they provide easily understood black-and-white answers to complex moral and ethical questions. Such groups are often led by a charismatic leader whom members idolize and depend on to do their thinking for them.

Religion can be used by patients as a defense during psychotherapy in order to avoid making changes in the way they relate to themselves and to other people—changes that are frightening but necessary for personal growth to take place. Religious beliefs may also block important psychodynamic insights and understandings that could help release patients from maladaptive patterns, lead to greater insight, and achieve greater intimacy in relationships with others. The religious person may become frustrated because he or she cannot forgive an individual and may feel guilty about it, turning to prayer or confession instead of pursuing the necessary therapy that could provide insight into why he or she is having trouble forgiving.

Because of the greater emotional and mental fragility of psychiatric patients and the greater amount of time spent with their MH therapists, relationships that develop are often more intense than would ordinarily develop with other HPs whom they contact about physical problems and with whom they spend relatively little time. The result is more intense "transference" reactions to their therapists, where the therapist is treated as if he or she were a parent figure or other influential person during childhood. The therapist, then, may have unusual power to influence the religious patient's beliefs (increasing the risk of coercion), or in contrast, the patient may resist suggestions by the therapist (as a parent figure), cloaking that resistance in religious explanations.

A therapist may likewise have "countertransference" reactions to patients because of the therapist's past relationships and religious experiences, and may experience repulsion or disgust with patients who are making poor moral decisions or refusing to live up to the religious therapist's high moral standards.[15] Alternatively, the nonreligious therapist may have the same negative reaction to a religious patient, whose beliefs are seen as neurotic or delusional.

In order for the therapist to help such patients, boundary issues related to religion become even more important. This is particularly true when the therapist is attempting to use religious or spiritual beliefs/activities in the therapeutic approach. Fragile patients may have difficulty separating their own religious beliefs from the religious beliefs of the therapist, and vice versa for therapists with strong religious beliefs. Religion, then, can become hopelessly entangled in the therapeutic relationship and lead to arguments or other therapeutically unhelpful interactions. Thus, it becomes imperative for MH specialists to be aware of the ways that religion can threaten the therapeutic alliance with patients and maintain clear and firm boundaries on where and how deep they go in addressing religious issues, especially if the MH specialist has no training in pastoral counseling.

Adherence to relationship boundaries is particularly important when the MH professional is performing insight-oriented psychotherapy. The MH professional must maintain the tightly defined relationship between patient and therapist so it can be used as a therapeutic tool. A MH professional is in danger of overstepping professional boundaries if he or she treats the patient in a way that encourages personal friendship or becomes personally involved with the patient or the patient's problems. Such over-involvement threatens to compromise the MH professional's objectivity, the development of the transference, and the MH professional's ability to use the therapeutic relationship to help the patient. Patients are usually unaware of such boundary issues and so will often test those boundaries by wanting to know more about the MH professional, the MH professional's family, where they live, and where they go on vacation (as in the popular movie *What About Bob?* with Bill Murray).

The patient may probe for personal information about the MH professional in order to form a personal relationship, but usually in the same maladaptive manner as the patient does with other people. It is often that maladaptive way of relating to others that has brought the patient in for treatment. The responsibility of the MH professional, then, is to maintain the therapeutic relationship and to enforce the boundaries in the relationship by not giving out personal information or fostering personal involvement with the patient. If the therapeutic approach being taken is purely supportive (providing emotional support to the patient), then rigid adherence to boundaries is less crucial—although still necessary to some extent to maintain objectivity, especially for MH professionals who are making treatment decisions.

Professional pastoral counselors have specific training on how to handle transference and countertransference problems related to religion, and often must go through therapy themselves to better understand how their own religious beliefs affect their view of the world, their relationships in it, and future relationships with patients. Professional healthcare chaplains may also have special training on spiritual issues in patients with severe emotional or mental health problems, but such training for chaplains is not universal.

WHAT SHOULD MENTAL HEALTH SPECIALISTS DO?

Despite these concerns, there are ways to sensibly integrate spirituality into the mental health care of patients, depending on how much pastoral training and experience the MH professional has. Many of the same principles for integrating spirituality into patient care described for medical HPs apply to mental health HPs. The least controversial of these is the spiritual history.

Spiritual History. Because of the close relationship between psychological, social, and spiritual issues, it is necessary for the MH professional (regardless of pastoral counseling experience) to take a thorough spiritual history as part of the initial evaluation of all psychiatric patients. The spiritual history will be more detailed and will take more time than with medical patients.

The MH spiritual history should gather information about the patient's religious background and experiences during childhood, adolescence, and adulthood (across the lifespan), and determine how religion has been used in the past and is being used in the present to cope with life problems. Of particular importance is inquiry about any past negative experiences with religion, including disappointments due to unanswered prayers, major losses, stressful events, or conflicts with clergy or other members of the congregation. Religious beliefs and activities (public and private) should be explored. Religion can be either a powerful coping behavior that relieves distress and provides profound comfort and stability or it can contribute to the psychopathology for which the patient is seeking help. The therapist's approach to the patient's religious beliefs (whether supportive, neutral, or challenging) will be directly influenced by the information learned.

Unlike in medical patients where any indication that the patient is not religious would stop further inquiry, the MH specialist may need to gently probe further to obtain a better understanding of the patient's prior negative experiences with religion. Situations that may have turned patients off to religion (such as sexual abuse by a religious authority or a traumatic event that altered their religious worldview) could be contributing to the patient's current psychiatric problems.[16] If the therapist meets firm resistance from the patient, then the topic should be tactfully dropped and approached at a later time after a therapeutic alliance has been established more firmly. The ultimate purpose is not to make the patient more or less religious, but rather to understand how this powerful cultural factor may be playing a role in the current problems for which the patient is seeking help (or could serve as a positive resource for the patient and the therapy).

Taking a spiritual history is particularly important for patients for whom psychotherapy or counseling is planned. The patient may have intensely held religious beliefs that could conflict with the type of psychotherapy planned and, if the therapist doesn't take the time to learn about these beliefs, then the therapy will not likely succeed. In their writings, *Prophets of Psychoheresy I and II,* Martin and Diedre Bobgan argue that Christians should avoid mental health care, especially psychotherapy.[17] Likewise, author Jay Adams, who has been hugely influential in the Christian evangelical community over the past twenty years (and is especially known for his best-selling book *Competent to Counsel*),[18] has criticized secular approaches to mental health care. Thus, negative attitudes toward traditional MH therapies are not uncommon in many devout Christian religious circles (and may likewise be present in other religious traditions as well). The same is true for patients for whom antidepressants or other psychiatric drugs are planned—religious attitudes may significantly affect drug compliance and treatment follow-up.[19]

The spiritual history should also gather information about whether the patient is a member of a religious or spiritual community, how active the patient is in that community, and how much support he or she receives from religious leaders and other members of the congregation. This will indicate how much social support the patient is receiving (besides support from family and non-church friends). The identity of the religious community will also help to determine if that community will encourage or discourage professional MH care. Level of the patient's involvement (frequency of attendance, participation in small groups, leadership or service activities) is also relevant because it indicates the extent to which the community is likely to influence the patient's decisions and behaviors.

Respect and Support Beliefs. As with other HPs, the MH specialist should always show respect for the patient's religious or spiritual beliefs, remembering that these beliefs often serve an important function in holding the patient's psyche together. Even bizarre or clearly pathological religious or spiritual beliefs should be handled with respect, and effort made to understand them without supporting or validating them. If after detailed examination the patient's beliefs do not appear obviously pathological and they appear to be helping the patient to cope, then the MH specialist may consider supporting them. Care should be taken, however, not to move too quickly from inquiry about and attempts to understand beliefs to supporting the beliefs. It is always better to take a respectful but neutral position until the MH specialist has a thorough understanding of the patient's symptoms, underlying personality structure, and psychopathology. Supporting religious beliefs and activities is most appropriate when the patient is dealing with situational stressors, which may include the difficult situation of being mentally ill.

Challenge Beliefs. If it becomes evident that religious or spiritual beliefs are contributing to or interwoven with the patient's psychopathology, then it is often best to maintain a respectful but neutral stance toward these beliefs (at least initially). If beliefs are being used defensively to avoid making important life changes or attitudinal shifts, then it may be necessary at some point to gently challenge those beliefs. Challenging religious beliefs, however, is a risky procedure, and should not be attempted until a firm therapeutic alliance has been established with the patient, a complete and thorough spiritual history has been taken, and multiple attempts over time made to change the patient's attitude and behavior in other therapeutic ways. It may be necessary to have a conversation with the patient's clergy or other religious leaders (or even include them in a therapy session, if the patient allows) before challenging the patient's religious beliefs. Advice from a trained MH chaplain or pastoral counselor can be invaluable here.

Before proceeding to challenge the patient's beliefs, as noted above, the MH specialist should have a thorough understanding of how his or her own religious beliefs could be influencing this decision. Countertransference problems should always must be recognized and dealt with by the MH provider before challenging a patient's religious beliefs. This is like doing brain surgery, and one false move can have disastrous consequences on both the therapeutic relationship and on the patient's mental stability (given the intensity of religious beliefs and their links to identity and meaning).

Prayer with Patients. Prayer with a religious patient, as noted in earlier chapters, can have a powerful positive therapeutic effect and strengthen the therapeutic alliance. This, however, is a more risky intervention that should not occur until the MH specialist knows the patient well and has a thorough understanding of the patient's religious or spiritual beliefs and prior experiences with religion. All of the conditions for praying with patients should be met as described previously—the patient should initiate the request, the patient's and the therapist's religious backgrounds should be similar, the therapist should ask what the patient wants prayer for, and so on.

Even if all the right conditions are present, there may still be some patients for whom prayer would be too intrusive, too personal, and may violate delicate boundaries that could interfere with the therapeutic relationship—particularly if the MH specialist says the prayer out loud with the patient. If the patient says the prayer, and the MH specialist is simply present and supportive, then there is less risk and the activity may provide useful information that can be used therapeutically. Prayer with MH patients, as with medical patients, should never be a matter of routine. The timing and intention should always be planned out as part of the therapeutic intervention, with clear goals in mind beforehand.

As with prayer in medical patients, the prayer said by the MH specialist should be short and supportive, using the language of the patient's faith tradition. Physical contact with the patient during prayer is a more delicate matter, and will depend on the MH specialist, the particular patient, age and gender, and therapeutic approach (medication vs. supportive vs. psychodynamic). Occasionally, holding hands with the patient during prayer may be permissible, but if there is any question at all that such a gesture will be misinterpreted by the patient, it is best to avoid physical contact entirely.

Consultation with or Referral to Clergy. Most MH specialists with minimal training can learn to take a spiritual history, be neutral or supportive with regard to patients' religious beliefs, and even pray with patients if done with caution and common sense. However, if specific training in pastoral counseling is lacking, the MH specialist may not want to challenge religious beliefs or integrate positive religious beliefs as part of a patient's therapy.

Consultation, referral, or joint therapy with trained clergy are other options. This is most appropriate when spiritual needs or conflicts come up during therapy, when religious issues are mixed up with the patient's psychopathology or are blocking progress, or when the therapist wishes to utilize the patient's religious resources in the treatment. In these circumstances, a non-pastorally trained MH professional may want to consult with a professional chaplain or pastoral counselor, or may choose to refer the patient to this person to handle the religious aspects of the case. Such consultation or referral should be done sooner rather than later if the MH specialist feels nervous, unprepared, or inexperienced with these matters. Referral, however, should not be made before a thorough spiritual history has been taken as described above, or before a therapeutic alliance has been established. Information from the spiritual history is necessary both for the MH specialist's treatment plan and for deciding on the particular pastoral care specialist to refer to (pastoral counselor, chaplain, other clergy).

Another option is to jointly treat a patient with a pastoral care specialist. Sessions with the patient may alternate between MH and pastoral care providers. Joint therapy, however, needs to be done carefully, so that secular and pastoral therapies are coordinated and not in conflict with one another, and communication must be close between treatment providers. This may not work with all patients, particularly fragile patients who may "split" secular and religious therapists, identifying one as the "good" and one as the "bad" parent figure and spur competition between the two.

SUMMARY AND CONCLUSIONS

Although many of the same principles apply to integrating spirituality into patient care for MH professionals as for medical professionals, there are important differences. Religious or spiritual issues are important for many patients dealing with emotional or mental problems and can be a tremendous resource for support and healing. Religion can also contribute to mental health problems in complex ways that may be difficult to sort out. MH specialists deal with psychologically fragile and unstable patients in whom religious or spiritual issues may be intricately interwoven with the psychopathology itself. Thus, a more thorough and detailed spiritual history is necessary than for a patient dealing only with medical issues. There are also boundary concerns that the MH specialist must be more conscious about, especially those related to transference and countertransference.

Respecting and, in some cases, supporting the religious beliefs and activities of patients may help with recovery and healing, as may prayer with patients. Integrating religious beliefs into therapy, however, requires more expertise, usually specific training in pastoral counseling or clinical pastoral education. Consultation with, referral to, or joint therapy with chaplains or pastoral counselors is indicated when there is a need to challenge religious beliefs or use religious beliefs as part of the therapy.

CHAPTER 12

A MODEL COURSE CURRICULUM

H ere I present a model course outline for integrating spirituality into patient care that can be used in
medical schools, medical or psychiatry residencies, psychology or counseling programs, nursing schools, schools
of social work, and in training programs for physical and
occupational therapists, physician assistants, nurse practitioners, and other health care professionals. Although
there is not a common curriculum currently used in any
HP training program, other models for medical curricula exist and the reader should be familiar with them.[1]
Below, I describe the ways that a spirituality course can
be *structured* within the existing curriculum, the *form*
that the course can take, and then describe the *content* of
what needs to be taught, using a spirituality curriculum
designed for medical schools as the initial example and
then showing how the basic content can be modified for
other HP curricula.

STRUCTURE AND TIMING

First, a decision has to be made on *how* the course will be structured within the existing curriculum. This will depend on how much overall time will be allowed for such a course, and when that time will be allowed. If little or no time is allowed, then a 60-minute lecture with 15 to 30 minutes for discussion will need to suffice. If enough time for a mini-course is allowed, then three or four 60- to 90-minute sessions may be possible. A full course would ideally involve at least ten 60- to 90-minute sessions.

A related issue is whether the course will be elective or required. If elective, only a handful of students are likely to attend, although these will be the students who really want to be there and more time will be available to treat the topic in greater depth. If the course is required, then all students will get some exposure to the topic, although the amount of material taught may be less. Currently, about 70 percent of spirituality courses in medical schools are required, which I think they ought to be.

Next, a decision must be made on *when* in the medical curriculum the course will be taught, and whether it should be taught only in a single block, separated into more than one block, or distributed throughout the curriculum. The structure of the medical curriculum to some extent determines the ideal time for presenting the spirituality curriculum to medical students. The first two years are often spent learning the basic/clinical sciences and being introduced to the human aspects of medicine. In the third year, medical students begin their clinical clerkships on the wards, learning the clinical material by actually doing it, and become responsible for patient care under the supervision of interns and residents. In the fourth year, more advanced clinical rotations will be taken and there will be time for a few electives. Some medical schools also require that a research project be completed in the third or fourth year.

The spirituality course could be taught in the first or second year of medical school, exposing medical students to these issues when they are just starting out. Another option is to teach the course in the fourth year along with a clinical rotation or a preceptorship with a physician working in the community. A third option is distributing the course throughout the four years of medical school. The spirituality course does not always need to be taught as a separate course; instead, it can be included as part of another course, such as the Medicine and Society course often taught in the first or second year. This course typically involves related topics on behavioral medicine, ethical issues, advanced care planning, doctor-patient communication, and complementary and alternative medicine. This does not mean simply doing what is already being done in these courses, but rather including specific content that explicitly addresses religious or spiritual issues.

If there is only time for a couple of lectures, then probably the worst time is during the first year of medical school, when students are being bombarded with the basic sciences and have no clinical experience with which to ground the material they learn on spirituality. Without clinical experience, it is difficult for students to grasp the meaning and relevancy of this topic that may be seen as the antithesis of "real science." However, if students are exposed to the material early on and it is reinforced by linking with actual cases during the clinical years, this will help the ideas to stick in their minds. Thus, if time and faculty are available and the dean is supportive, integrating it throughout the four-year curriculum is ideal, with the initial course taught in the first or second year and the concepts explicitly reinforced and modeled during the remaining two years when students are caring for patients.

FORM

The form that a spirituality curriculum takes can greatly vary, and it is probably wise to include as many different ways of presenting the material as possible. The available forms in order of low to high impact are: (1) reading an article/s from the medical literature; (2) attending a lecture (no discussion); (3) attending a lecture with a discussion; (4) listening to a case presentation followed by a discussion; (5) exposure to a live patient with questions from the class and later discussion; (6) faculty modeling within clinical settings; and (7) role-playing.

Articles. As with most medical training, students are often given seminal articles to read from the medical literature on topics they are studying. This is one of the least effective ways of learning but better than nothing and uses up virtually no time from the medical curriculum. Student may then be asked to give an oral report on the article to their peers, which will add value to the learning experience.

Lecture. Lectures are important because they can convey large amounts of information in a relatively short time. They are better than reading an article, because there is a live person speaking and hopefully engaging the audience through sight, sound, and personal interaction. Of course, for this modality to be successful, the speaker must be engaging.

Lecture with Discussion. Adding time for discussion after the lecture engages the students further and forces them to think and become involved with the topic. The speaker, however, must be very knowledgeable about the topic in order to handle all sorts of questions, and be able to moderate the discussion and group dynamics that ensue.

Presentation of a Case. Holding a case conference, where one of the students presents an actual case to the group that involves religious or spiritual issues, can be very effective learning, since students view cases as more clinically relevant and "stories" are always remembered better than facts. The case conference should include ample time for questions and discussion, allowing other students to get involved and deeper aspects of the topic to be explored.

Presentation of Live Patient. One of the most effective ways of presenting material is to have a live patient come to a conference room or lecture auditorium and describe his or her current experience of grappling with illness and the role that religious/spiritual beliefs and practices play to help him or her cope, derive meaning, and experience hope. The more dramatic the case and the more expressive the patient, the better. A student or faculty member first presents the case to the group. The patient then appears and tells his or her story. This is then followed by questions from students directly to the patient, with faculty moderating the process to clarify and make it easier on the patient. The patient then leaves the room, and a discussion follows.

Faculty Modeling. Here, faculty model taking a spiritual history or otherwise interacting with patients over spiritual matters in a clinical setting. This may take place on the hospital wards during medical rounds or in the outpatient clinics. A student may spend a month in a preceptorship with a clinician in the community who regularly addresses spiritual issues as part of his or her practice. This is one of the most effective forms of learning, because it involves seeing a seasoned clinician in action, direct experience of results, and repetition, and may even involve student practice (depending on the particular patient and the comfort level of the clinician).

Role-playing. Students may take turns role-playing patient and doctor. This works best for taking a spiritual history, supporting beliefs, and deciding on whether to refer to a chaplain (with a third student playing the chaplain, or having a student chaplain play this role). Role-playing, while a bit awkward when being done with fellow students, will help to significantly ease the discomfort involved in doing this with patients. Since discomfort is one of the main barriers that prevent physicians from addressing spiritual issues, role-playing and practice should be central to any well-rounded spirituality curriculum.

In summary, a course should be given designated time to teach issues specifically related to religion and spirituality. This course will start with an initial series of classes as an introduction, and then concepts will be applied and reinforced throughout the four years of medical school, timed so that they are relevant to what students are learning in other areas. It will include all of the above forms of teaching—articles, lectures, discussions, case presentations, faculty modeling, and role-playing. That is the ideal, and in real life, where most medical curricula are already packed to their limits, one takes whatever one can get.

CONTENT

The content of the spirituality curriculum is critical in determining what students will take away from the often brief exposure to this topic. The order of presenting material is also important. Below, I describe a ten-session model curriculum that will need to be adapted to the time and setting available. This ten-session course should ideally be taught in the first or second year and individual components of the course reemphasized and elaborated on at appropriate times in sync with material taught during the remaining years; alternatively, the individual sessions could be taught at different times during the four-year medical curriculum. The content presented below follows the main chapters of this book, *Spirituality in Patient Care* (SPC). Each session will take 60–90 minutes.

Session 1. Introduction to topic. Format: lecture and discussion. Content: A broad overview of spirituality and medicine should be presented, including a historical perspective, discussion of definitions (spirituality, religion, humanism), description of patients' spiritual needs and who is available to address them, brief description of each of the remaining nine sessions, and discussion of what is expected of students to successfully complete the course (including attendance and participation). Remainder of time should be allowed for student questions, clarifications, and discussion. Handout material to be read by next class: SPC introduction and chapter 1, along with a review article.[2]

Session 2. Why address spirituality in patient care? Format: case presentation followed by lecture and discussion. Content: Briefly present case, and then review the six reasons why spirituality should be addressed by physicians (defer discussion of research on religion and health to next session). End lecture with data on how patients feel, how physicians feel, and what physicians are currently doing with regard to identifying or addressing patients' spiritual needs. Use remainder of time for discussion. Handout material to be read by next class: choose a combination of best original research on mental health,[3] physical health,[4] and pro/con review articles.[5]

Session 3. The research. Format: lecture and discussion. Content: Lecture should cover three areas: (1) examine religion/spirituality and mental health; (2) discuss mind-body relationships (psychoneuroimmunology and stress-related cardiovascular system changes); and (3) describe a model of how religion/spirituality could affect physical health, and present research on religion/spirituality and physical health. This is a lot of material to cover, but time is also needed for discussion (pros and cons regarding quality of existing research). Handout material to be read by next class: article about a religious patient.[6]

Session 4. The patient's perspective. Format: live case presentation, questions, and discussion. Content: Identify a patient who is seriously ill, articulate, deeply religious, and using his or her beliefs or support from a faith community to help him or her cope. The patient may be an inpatient or an outpatient. Students should be given ample time to question the patient directly, although faculty may need to assist by rephrasing questions to make it easier on the patient. End with a discussion after the patient leaves. This can be the most powerful of all the sessions if the right patient is chosen. Handout material to be read by next class: SPC chapters 2 and 7, spiritual history[7] and clinical applications[8] articles.

Session 5. How to include spirituality. Format: lecture and role-playing. Content: Describe how to take a spiritual history, patient-centered approach, showing respect for and supporting the patient's beliefs, and praying with patient. During this session, the role of the professional chaplain should be discussed, paying particular attention to the training of the board-certified chaplain, the tasks of the chaplain in the health care setting (chapter 7), and when to refer patients to chaplains. Lecture should be followed by questions from students to clarify the "how-to's." If there is time left, students should be broken up into pairs for practice taking a spiritual history on each other. Handout material to be read by next class: SPC chapter 3 and Hastings Center Report article.[9]

Session 6. When to include spirituality. Format: lecture, discussion, and role-playing. Content: Lecture will focus on the timing of spiritual histories, the conditions for praying with patients, and when a chaplain referral is necessary, with discussion to follow. If there was insufficient time in Session 5 for role-playing, this might be a good time for students to practice these techniques. Handout material to be read by next class: SPC chapter 4 and article on clinical trial involving spiritual history.[10]

Session 7. Consequences of including spirituality. Format: case presentation, lecture, and discussion. Content: Case and lecture should focus on what might result when physician takes a spiritual history, supports beliefs of patient, engages in religious activities with patients (prayer), or refers patients to chaplains. Both positive and negative consequences should be discussed. This will help students understand the benefits of addressing spirituality and also some of the negative responses that they may run into. Handout material to be read by next class: SPC chapter 5, Annals of Internal Medicine article on boundaries,[11] and legal update on church-state separation issues.[12]

Session 8. Barriers and boundaries. Format: lecture and discussion. Content: Lecture should focus on barriers that physicians say prevent them from taking a spiritual history or communicating with patients about the spiritual aspects of medical care. For this session, it is particularly important to have plenty of time for discussion. May also wish to expose students to church-state separation controversies. Discussing issues related to (a) patient "choice," (b) patient "isolation" from religious support tailored to medical illness, and (c) need for the physician's focus to be on secular goals (i.e., the patient's health, not religion) will help students avoid future problems in this area. Handout material to be read by next class: SPC chapter 6, NEJM article by Sloan[13] and brief letter to the editor in response.[14]

Session 9. Possibility of harm. Form: case presentation, lecture, and discussion. Content: Case and lecture should focus on the potential harm that could result from physicians taking a spiritual history, supporting patients' beliefs, participating in religious activities such as prayer with patients, or referring to chaplains. The purpose of discussing the possibility of "harm" is so that the physician will be fully prepared for any situation that may arise (no matter how unlikely). Again, plenty of time should be reserved for discussion among students. Handout material to be read by next class: SPC chapter 13.

Session 10. Addressing spirituality in a multicultural, multi-religious setting. Format: Case presentation, lecture, and discussion. Content: Case should be of a devoutly religious patient from a religious background that is completely different from that of most students. In a pluralistic health care setting, physicians are likely to encounter patients from many different religious traditions. Students should have a general knowledge of how different religious traditions deal with birth and contraception, diet, illness, death, and dying, so that accommodations can be made to show respect for these traditions. This is also a good time to reinforce chaplains as an important resource, given their knowledge about and training on how to address the needs of patients from diverse religious backgrounds.

After completing these ten sessions, medical students and residents should have confidence in their ability to appropriately and sensitively address spiritual issues in patient care. They should understand why communication with patients about spiritual issues is important, how to go about doing this, when to do so, what boundaries they should not cross, what the consequences might be, and how to handle different situations. They should also understand the roles of professional chaplains, pastoral counselors, and clergy, and how they can assist the physician in this area. The only thing left, then, is for students to actually begin doing it—integrating spirituality into the way they care for patients.

ADAPTING THE COURSE FOR OTHER HPS

Nursing, social work, and physical and occupational therapy programs can easily adapt the above model curriculum to meet the needs of their students. The research reviewed in chapters 8, 9, and 10 makes it clear that the vast majority of HPs in these disciplines are not receiving adequate training to address the spiritual needs of their patients. Even though the above curriculum is directed towards physicians, the content is basic for the training of all HPs so that they can screen for spiritual needs, determine what they can and cannot address, and know when to refer patients to spiritual care specialists. Bear in mind that only about one in ten physicians regularly takes a spiritual history or addresses these issues. This means that if patients' spiritual needs are going to be identified and addressed, in nine out of ten cases, someone other than a physician will have to do it.

Nurses. As mentioned earlier, if the physician does not do it, then the task of taking a spiritual history naturally falls to nurses, especially if spiritual needs are to be identified early enough during hospitalization so that they can be addressed by chaplains before discharge. However, the nursing curriculum is just as packed as the medical curriculum, especially as nurses training becomes shorter and shorter in attempts to make up for the growing nursing shortage we are facing as the population ages. However, because of the JCAHO requirement and the fact that chaplains are not able to see all patients to do spiritual assessments, it is imperative that nursing education include something about spirituality in the required curriculum. The content of that training should focus on why, how, and when to conduct a spiritual history, where to document this, when to refer to chaplains, and the health-related traditions of different religious groups. This will at least meet the minimum requirement. I recommend sessions 2, 5, 6 and 10 above; assigned reading of SPC chapters 1–3, 5, 7, 8 and 13; and supplemented with readings from one of the major "spirituality in nursing" texts.[15]

Social Workers. As emphasized previously, if nurses do not screen patients for spiritual needs, then this task falls to the social worker. The social work curriculum has no more free time to devote to learning these tasks than does the nursing curriculum. And social workers have an additional role that nurses do not have. Ensuring that spiritual needs are adequately addressed at the time of discharge and developing a discharge spiritual care plan (with the chaplain) are other social work tasks. Social workers need to ensure that any incompletely addressed spiritual needs of patients are conveyed to the community where the patient will be living (home, nursing home, or rehabilitation setting) so that pastoral care follow-up can be arranged. Thus, social workers not only need to know how to take and document a spiritual history (if not already done), but also must work with chaplains to develop a discharge plan that addresses the spiritual needs uncovered. This will require a short course in the social work curriculum addressing the why, how, and when of addressing spiritual needs, the role of chaplains and pastoral counselors, the health-related practices of different religions, developing a spiritual care discharge plan, and working with faith communities. I recommend sessions 2, 5, 6, and 10 above; assigned reading of SPC chapters 1–3, 5, 7, 9 and 13; and articles from the social work literature.[16]

Physical and Occupational Therapy. As noted in chapter 10, physical and occupational therapists are involved in enabling patients to regain physical functioning and independent living. Spiritual and religious beliefs play an important role in motivating religious patients to regain their function so that they can once more engage in religious and altruistic activities that give live meaning, purpose, and joy. Training on how and when to take a spiritual history, pray with patients if requested, and work with chaplains to address patients' spiritual needs should be a part of any holistic training program in the rehabilitation specialties. I recommend sessions 2, 5, 6, and 10; assigned reading of SPC chapters 1–3, 5, 7, 10 and 13; and articles from the rehabilitation literature.[17]

SUMMARY AND CONCLUSIONS

In this chapter, the structure, timing, and form of a spirituality curriculum were discussed, and the content of a ten-session model curriculum was described. Although the initial curriculum was developed with reference to medical students and residents, I demonstrated ways that the curriculum could be adapted for the training of nurses, social workers, and rehabilitation therapists. The goal is to have a single, consistent curriculum implemented across the health care specialties that takes advantage of the unique training, strengths, and position of each health care profession to ensure that patients' spiritual needs are met in whatever setting patients find themselves.[18]

CHAPTER 13

INFORMATION ON SPECIFIC RELIGIONS

This chapter provides basic information that health professionals need to know about the health practices of patients from various religious traditions that may influence their health care. The information presented here is not exhaustive, and many religious traditions have not been included because of limited space. The focus is on major religious traditions that HPs are most likely to encounter during their daily work with patients. What is presented here is a condensed version of information contained in chapters by Verna B. Carson in *Spiritual Dimensions of Nursing*.[1] Information has also been taken from a comprehensive text prepared by Sue Wintz and Earl Cooper for the Association of Professional Chaplains.[2] The reader should turn to these resources for details about the care practices of religious traditions that are not covered in this brief synopsis. Remember, though, when there is any doubt about a religious practice related to health care, the HP should always respectfully ask the patient or family about the religious practices that are important to them.

WESTERN RELIGIOUS TRADITIONS

CHRISTIANITY

Christianity is the largest religion in the world, with over 2.1 billion adherents, and is the largest religion in the United States, comprising 82 percent of the total population.[3]

Catholicism

Roman Catholic

Birth and Contraception

- Infant baptism is mandatory.
- Emergency baptism required for sick newborns, stillbirths, and aborted fetuses.
- Priest must do baptism; if emergent, and priest not available, anyone can baptize: pour warm water on infant's head saying, "I baptize you in the name of the Father, of the Son, and of the Holy Spirit" (record all information on chart and notify priest and family).
- Birth control is prohibited except by abstinence or natural family planning; Catholics may or may not follow this church teaching, so ask patients about their views and refer any questions regarding this to a priest or refer patients to a support group of the church that instructs couples on birth control.
- Abortion and sterilization are prohibited unless there is a clear medical reason to do so.

Diet

• Before receiving the sacrament of Holy Communion (Eucharist), patient must abstain from solid food and alcohol for a minimum of fifteen minutes (if possible); medicine is permitted and, if the person is in danger of death, no fast is required.

• Obligatory fasting is waived during hospitalization, although some Catholics may still abstain from eating meat on Ash Wednesday and all Fridays during Lent, or all Fridays throughout the year (offer fish).

Death, Dying, and Healing

• Any person who is sick and desires the sacrament of Anointing of the Sick may receive it from a priest, who anoints the forehead with oil and says a prayer; the purpose of the sacrament is for complete healing and strength to cope.

• Prior to 1963, Anointing of the Sick (or Extreme Unction) was done only if death was imminent, and many Catholics still think of the sacrament in this way.

• If sudden death occurs, Anointing of Sick may also be done shortly after death.

• HP should record in patient's record that Anointing of Sick has been done by the priest.

• Catholics are expected to participate in Anointing of Sick, Eucharist, and the sacrament of reconciliation (penance, confession) before death; body should not be shrouded until Anointing of Sick is completed.

• All body parts that can be recognized as a human part should be buried or cremated.

• Donation of organs and acceptance of transplants are acceptable.

Miscellaneous Rituals/Customs

• Religious objects important to Catholics are rosary beads (for saying prayers), medals of saints (that may be pinned to pillow or gown, worn around neck), and statues of saints or the Virgin Mary (that may be placed on bedside table); health care professional should safeguard these items.

Eastern Orthodox

Birth and Contraception

• A baby must be baptized within forty days after birth; sprinkling or immersion into water is the usual method (although if not possible, the baptism can be performed by moving the baby in the air in the sign of the cross); an ordained priest or a deacon must be the person who performs the baptism.

• Birth control is not allowed (although ask the patient, since adherence to this will vary).

• Abortion is not allowed except in medically necessary circumstances.

Diet

• Fasting is important and required; must refrain from eating meat and dairy products on Wednesday and Friday during Lent and on other holy days, although hospitalized patients are exempt if fasting could be harmful.

Death, Dying, and Healing

• If the patient desires, a priest may administer Anointing of the Sick in the patient's room for healing (different from Last Rites).

• When a person dies, he or she is required to receive Last

Rites, which is done by an ordained priest while the patient is conscious (preferably).

- If Russian Orthodox, autopsy or organ donation is discouraged.
- Euthanasia is discouraged in all circumstances.
- Cremation is discouraged.

Miscellaneous Rituals/Customs

- Sacraments are very important (Eucharist, Anointing of Sick, Last Rites).
- If the patient desires, HP may notify priest to administer Holy Eucharist.
- Major holidays are different for the Eastern Orthodox: Christmas is celebrated on January 7 and New Year's on January 14.

Protestant Denominations

Episcopal (Anglican)

Birth and Contraception

- A baby is baptized shortly after birth, which is urgent if the infant is serious ill and may die; notify a priest to administer baptism if there is time, although in an emergency, non-clergy may baptize an infant.
- No strict rules about contraception.

Diet

- No strict dietary rules, although some may choose to not eat meat on Fridays, and some may fast before taking the Holy Eucharist (although not required).

Death, Dying, and Healing

- Anointing of the Sick is done if death is imminent, but is not required; if a patient wishes, this sacrament may be administered whether the patient is dying or not.
- No particular rites surrounding death (except anointing just before death).

Miscellaneous Rituals/Customs

- Holy Eucharist/Communion is important in this tradition, and should be administered by an Episcopal priest or a deacon.
- Confession is practiced (although not required), and clergy should be notified if a patient wants this.

Lutheran

Birth and Contraception

- Infants are baptized six to eight weeks after birth.
- Stillborn infants are not usually baptized.
- Adults are also baptized, which may involve sprinkling, pouring, or water immersion.
- No strict rules about contraception.

Diet

- No special dietary practices

Death, Dying, and Healing

- If requested, sick (particularly dying) patients are anointed with oil by the minister.
- On death, a Commendation of the Dying service is held, depending on the wishes of the patient or family.

Miscellaneous Rituals/Customs

- Holy Eucharist/Communion is important; notify clergy if the patient requests it.

Methodist

Birth and Contraception

- Baptism may be requested by parents if an infant is sick.
- No strict rules about contraception.

Diet

- No special dietary practices.

Death, Dying, and Healing

- Anointing of the Sick is performed by clergy (prayer and oil) for healing.
- Reading of scripture and prayer may be important for family before and after death.
- Organ donation after death is encouraged.

Miscellaneous Rituals/Customs

- Holy Communion/Eucharist may be requested if the patient is seriously ill or undergoing surgery.

Presbyterian

Birth and Contraception

- Infants are baptized by pouring or sprinkling by the pastor; baptism by immersion may be practiced with adults.
- No strict rules about contraception.

Diet

- No special dietary practices.

Death, Dying, and Healing

- On a patient's death, the family may request their pastor or an elder to pray and read scripture.

Miscellaneous Rituals/Customs

- Holy Communion/Eucharist is administered by pastor if patient requests it.

United Church of Christ

Birth and Contraception

- Infant and adult baptism are practiced.

Diet

- No special dietary practices.

Death, Dying, and Healing

- Patient may request prayer if dying.

Miscellaneous Rituals/Customs

- Holy Communion/Eucharist may be requested by the patient and is administered by a minister.

Baptist (27 different groups)

Birth and Contraception

- Infants are not baptized.

Diet

- Total abstinence from alcohol is required by many groups.

Death, Dying, and Healing

- When near death, patient often requests the presence of a pastor, who may provide prayer, scripture reading, and counselling.
- It is important that the patient confess Jesus Christ as his or her personal Lord and Savior before he or she dies, if this has not already been done (many believe that this is required for admittance to heaven).

Miscellaneous Rituals/Customs

- If the patient desires, clergy will administer Holy Eucharist.
- The Bible is considered the word of God and the ultimate authority, and the patient may want scripture passages read to him or her by family members or members of the church (or by health professionals).

Assemblies of God (Pentecostal)

Birth and Contraception

- No infant baptism, although there may be a dedication.
- Baptism is performed by complete immersion in water after the person has received Jesus Christ as his or her personal Lord and Savior once he or she is able to consciously and meaningfully make this decision.
- No strict rules regarding contraception, although abortion is strongly opposed.

Diet

• Abstinence from alcohol and smoking is emphasized (although not strictly forbidden).

Death, Dying, and Healing

• Belief in divine healing is strong, and many patients (or family members) will want this; anointing of the sick may be administered by clergy or a layperson.

• After death, there are no special practices, although it is very important that the person confess Jesus Christ as his or her personal Lord and Savior before he or she dies (many believe that this is required for admittance to heaven).

Miscellaneous Rituals/Customs

• The patient may desire Holy Eucharist/Communion; administered by clergy (or by laypersons in some denominations).

• The Bible is considered the word of God and the ultimate authority, and patient may want scripture passages read to him or her by family members or members of the church (or by health professionals).

• Prayer is very important, and time should be allowed for this; prayer may include "speaking in tongues."

Mennonite

Birth and Contraception

• No infant baptism is practiced; a baby may be dedicated if the parents wish.

• Ask about rules concerning contraception.

Diet

• No special dietary practices, although the use of alcohol is strongly discouraged.

Death, Dying, and Healing

• Contact a minister for prayer if a patient is seriously ill, or for the family after a patient's death (ask family).

• Patients may request anointing with oil for healing.

• Holy Eucharist/Communion is offered twice yearly, with foot-washing ceremony (patient or family may request this if a patient is serious ill).

Miscellaneous Rituals/Customs

• Women may wear head coverings during hospitalization.

Church of the Brethren

Birth and Contraception

• No infant baptism, but there may be a dedication service.

Death, Dying, and Healing

• Anointing of the sick is performed by clergy, and is important; this is done for physical healing as well as for emotional comfort.

• When a patient is dying, clergy should be requested for support and prayer.

Miscellaneous Rituals/Customs

• Holy Eucharist/Communion will be administered in the hospital by clergy if a patient requests it.

Church of the Nazarene

Birth and Contraception

• A baby may be dedicated or baptized, depending on the parents' wishes.

Diet

• Alcohol and smoking are not allowed; no other dietary concerns.

Death, Dying, and Healing

• Medical treatment and divine healing are both encouraged.
• Cremation is acceptable.
• Full-term stillborn infants should be buried.

Miscellaneous Rituals/Customs

• Believers' baptism is important.
• Holy Eucharist/Communion will be administered by clergy at the patient's request.

Disciples of Christ

Birth and Contraception

• No infant baptism, but a dedication service is usually held after birth; baptism is by immersion in water after the age of accountability (when able to make conscious decisions).

Diet

• No special practices.

Death, Dying, and Healing

• No special practices after death.

Miscellaneous Rituals/Customs

• Holy Eucharist (Communion) is important, and the patient may request it from a member of the clergy.

• Clergy or church members are urged to visit to meet patients' spiritual needs.

Salvation Army

Birth and Contraception

• An infant dedication service is practiced.

• Abortion is opposed unless medically necessary.

• No other rules against medication or surgery or contraception.

Diet

• No special practices.

Death, Dying, and Healing

• At the time of illness or death, notify the local officer in charge of the Salvation Army Corps, if requested.

Miscellaneous Rituals/Customs

• Members are called soldiers.

• Make a Bible available to the patient, since this is important.

Seventh-day Adventist

Birth and Contraception

• No infant baptism; dedication services may be held after birth.

• No restrictions on birth control.

• Abortion only allowed in case of rape, incest, or danger to the mother's life.

Diet

- Healthy lifestyle and eating habits are strongly encouraged.
- Alcohol, smoking, coffee, and tea are prohibited.
- Many are vegetarians, and almost all avoid pork.

Death, Dying, and Healing

- After death, no special practices are observed.
- Anointing with oil is administered by clergy, whether or not a patient is dying.
- Euthanasia is not permitted.
- Autopsy, donation of organs, and receipt of organs are all acceptable.

Miscellaneous Rituals/Customs

- The Sabbath is practiced on Saturday rather than Sunday.
- The Bible is important and a copy should be made available to patients.
- Holy Eucharist/Communion is administered by clergy if the patient requests it.
- Use of hypnosis is discouraged (although this varies).
- No restrictions on medications, blood, vaccines, or surgeries.
- Ask before administering narcotics or stimulants (and identify these to the patient).

Religious Society of Friends (Quaker)

Baptism and Contraception

- Baptism and Holy Eucharist/Communion are not usually practiced, but some Quakers may baptize with water; health professionals should inquire about particular beliefs/practices.
- Names of infants are recorded in a special book during the Quaker meeting.

Diet

• No particular dietary practices

Death, Dying, and Healing

• A burial ceremony may not be practiced, but follow the wishes of the patient or family.

Christian Science

Birth and Contraception

• Birth is assisted by a physician or a midwife (ask the patient).
• No baptism is performed.
• No rules about family planning or birth control.

Diet

• Alcohol and smoking are not permitted; coffee or tea are often refused.
• Many follow no dietary restrictions.

Death, Dying, and Healing

• After death, an autopsy is usually refused except if legally required.
• Donation of organs is not usually done, although there are no requirements in this regard.
• Euthanasia is forbidden.

Miscellaneous Rituals/Customs

• Sickness is believed to be due to lack of harmony between mind and body.
• May not seek medical care (except for birth), depending on how closely the teachings of Christian Science are followed.

- May refuse drugs or medical or surgical procedures.

- Many are not entirely opposed to medical treatment, and most will receive whatever medical treatment is required by law; always ask patients what kinds of treatment they will allow.

- Will allow a surgeon to splint a fracture.

- May refuse psychotherapy or hypnotism.

- May seek exemptions from vaccination, but they follow the law in this regard.

- Christian Science nonmedical facilities are available for those needing nursing care to facilitate healing.

- The *Christian Science Journal* publishes a list of qualified health providers called Christian Science practitioners (nonmedical).

- When hospitalized, time should be provided for prayer and scripture study.

- A Christian Science practitioner may be requested and should be allowed; the practitioner will practice spiritual healing, which is different from medical or psychological treatments.

Jehovah's Witness

Birth and Contraception

- Infant baptism is not practiced; complete-immersion baptism is performed with adults.

- Birth control is permitted.

- Abortion and artificial insemination (from a donor) are not permitted.

Diet

- Alcohol and smoking are not allowed.

- No other dietary rules except to avoid food that contains blood.

Death, Dying, and Healing

• Euthanasia is not permitted.

• After death, autopsy is permitted if legally required, but no body parts should be removed.

• Cremation or regular burial is acceptable.

• Organ donation is permitted.

Miscellaneous Rituals/Customs

• Organ transplants are allowed, but the organs must be washed with a non-blood solution before surgery.

• Blood transfusions are not allowed, and some patients are willing to die rather than accept blood (always check with the patient or surrogate decision maker about this).

• Will accept alternatives to blood, such as plasma expanders, use of autologous transfusions or autotransfusion (although some restrictions may be placed on these); consult with the local Jehovah's Witnesses hospital liaison committee.

• Medications made from blood products may not be permitted.

• For unconscious patients, check for medic-alert cards concerning blood transfusions.

• May not celebrate the usual Christian holidays.

THE CHURCH OF JESUS CHRIST OF LATTER-DAY SAINTS (MORMON)

Birth and Contraception

• Baptism by immersion is done at age eight or older (the age of accountability); it is not usually administered in a hospital setting.

• Abortion is not allowed unless the mother's life is in danger.

- Contraception is not allowed unless the physical or emotional health of the woman is at stake.
- Artificial insemination is acceptable if between husband and wife.

Diet

- Smoking, caffeine containing drinks (coffee and tea), or alcohol are not permitted.
- Mormons eat meat sparingly, but encourage vegetarian foods.
- 24-hour fasting (food and water) is encouraged once a month, although waived for the sick.

Death, Dying, and Healing

- Anointing of the sick, by giving a special blessing through a laying on of hands, may be done before and after hospital admission (two elders are usually required for this ritual blessing).
- After death, they encourage burial of the body (cremation is discouraged); notify a church elder to assist the family. This person may also help to dress the body in special clothes.
- Euthanasia or assisted suicide is not permitted.
- Autopsy and organ donation are permitted.
- No restrictions on medications, vaccinations, or blood products.

Miscellaneous Rituals/Customs

- A sacred garment may be worn by Mormons; it should only be removed in an emergency and should not be cut or damaged, but treated as a religious object.
- Mormon patients need time for prayer and reading scripture.

• Family visiting very important, and should be allowed/encouraged.

• Holy Eucharist/Communion (the Sacrament) may be requested by the patient, and a member of church's priesthood should be called.

UNITARIAN UNIVERSALISM

Birth and Contraception

• Dedication only; infant baptism is usually not practiced.
• Birth control is strongly encouraged.
• Abortion is allowed.

Diet

• No restrictions.

Death, Dying, and Healing

• After death, cremation is often preferred.
• Organ donation and transplantation are allowed.

JUDAISM

Judaism is the second largest religion in the United States (nearly 4 million or 2% of population) after Christianity. About 10 percent of American Jews are estimated to be Orthodox. However, Orthodox synagogues represent 40 percent of all U.S. synagogues, Reform synagogues about 26 percent, and Conservative synagogues about 23 percent.[4]

Orthodox and Some Conservative Branches

Birth and Contraception

• For male babies, ritual circumcision occurs eight days after birth, although it may be postponed due to poor health; circumcision is performed by a *mohel* (a person of the Jewish faith who is ordained to do circumcision under guidelines of the Jewish religion).

• A baby is named on the eighth day after birth, so health professionals should be cautious when referring to a baby before he or she is named.

• Women are in a state of impurity during menstrual periods or after childbirth; a husband will not touch his wife during this time (or even her bed). When the appropriate time comes, women will purify themselves by bathing in a pool called a *mikvah* (a ritual bath used for immersion during a purification ceremony).

• An Orthodox Jewish male will not touch any female other than his wife, daughters, or mother.

• Artificial birth control is not encouraged; vasectomy is not allowed.

• Abortion is allowed only to save the life of the mother.

• A miscarried fetus is usually buried, since it is considered a human being.

Diet

• Kosher dietary rules are followed more or less strictly:

1. No pork, ham, bacon, or any pork by-products, or any food prepared using pork or in contact with pork; no shellfish.

2. No mixing of milk and meat as part of a meal (including use of separate cooking utensils for milk and meat); if both are served during a meal, dairy products should be served first and then meat products.

3. No consumption of any animal products where the animal has not been slaughtered according to Jewish law.

4. A 24-hour fast is required during Yom Kippur (September 22 in 2007; depends on the Jewish calendar), although this requirement may be waived for medical reasons.

5. No leavened products (foods with yeast) may be eaten during eight days of Passover (April 12–20 in 2006, April 2–10 in 2007; depends on the Jewish calendar).

6. A time of quiet should be provided to say a prayer before and after meals.

• Wine may be used as part of religious ritual.

Death, Dying, and Healing

• Euthanasia or assisted suicide is forbidden by Orthodox Jews, and all life-support measures are aggressively pursued; however, ineffective medical treatments may not need to be continued.

• Visiting by family and friends prior to a patient's death is considered a religious duty; the Torah or Psalms may be read.

• The Jewish belief is that the person should have someone with him or her at the time when the soul leaves the body; thus, family or friends should be allowed to stay with Jewish patients who may be at risk for dying.

• When a person dies, the body should be untouched for 8–30 minutes, and then left alone until buried. Burial needs to occur within twenty-four hours (without flowers). Health professionals should not touch or wash the body; only an Orthodox Jew (or Jewish burial society) can care for the body. If necessary, nursing staff may provide routine care for the body, but should wear gloves (check with family about this). Mirrors in the room should be covered.

- On the Sabbath, Jews cannot handle a corpse.
- Funeral homes may need to be "approved"; cremation is not usually allowed.
- Autopsies are not usually allowed; if required, then all body parts must remain with the body (even without autopsy, all body parts must be buried with the body, even if limbs are lost in accident or surgery).
- A fetus must be buried.
- A seven-day mourning period is required for family, who must stay at home.
- Donor organ transplants are generally not allowed, but may be permitted in some circumstances with rabbinical consent (rules regarding organ donation may vary).

Miscellaneous Rituals/Customs

- Patients should not be touched by health care providers of the opposite sex.
- For Orthodox Jews, shaving should not be done with a razor, but with scissors or an electric shaver (the blade should not contact the skin).
- Orthodox men must wear skull caps at all times; women must cover their hair after marriage (some may wear wigs).
- Conservative Jews wear head coverings only during acts of worship or prayer.
- The Jewish Sabbath begins at sunset on Friday and ends at sunset on Saturday. On the Sabbath, Orthodox Jews do not ride in a car, smoke, turn on lights, handle money, use a telephone, or watch TV. Tests and surgery should be scheduled around the Sabbath as possible.
- Health care professional should provide time and quiet for prayer (required).

Reform

Birth and Contraception

- Favor ritual circumcision, but not required.
- No rules against touching women.

Diet

- Usually do not observe a kosher diet.

Death, Dying, and Healing

- Encourage the use of life support without heroic measures.
- Cremation is allowed, but families are encouraged to bury ashes in a Jewish cemetery.
- Donations of organs or transplantation are allowed if a rabbi gives permission.

Miscellaneous Rituals/Customs

- Generally, pray without head coverings or skull caps.
- Usually worship in temples on Friday evenings, but no strict rules.

ISLAM

Islam is the second largest religion in the world, with over 1 billion adherents, and is the third largest religion in the United States, with estimates of 1.6 to 5 million adherents, second only to Judaism.[5]

Birth and Contraception

- Allow women to wear their own gowns so they can cover the entire body, including the head.

- Prefer female staff to care for Muslim women (see below).
- Bathe baby immediately after birth, before giving to the mother.
- Father (or mother if no father) whispers a prayer in an infant's ears after birth.
- No baptism is practiced.
- Premature baby of at least 130 days gestation is treated as infant.
- Circumcision after birth is encouraged for males.
- During menstruation and forty days after birth, women are exempt from prayer, since this is a time of cleansing.
- Abortion is not allowed except in cases of grave risk to the mother's life.
- Contraception is discouraged by conservative Muslims, although Islamic law permits contraception.

Diet

- No alcohol, pork (bacon, ham), or shellfish is allowed; may eat beef, poultry, and lamb only if it prepared by a Muslim according to Islamic law, so patients may refuse to eat hospital food and insist that food be brought from home.
- Only vegetable oil is used in preparing foods.
- No restrictions on fish, vegetables, dairy products, or fruit.
- During the ninth month of the Muslim calendar (Ramadan), fasting from food and drink is expected from dawn to dusk; the sick, travellers, nursing mothers, and small children may be exempted.
- The first three days of the tenth month are marked by feasting (Eid-al-Fitr).

Death, Dying, and Healing

- Blood, medications, vaccinations, amputations, organ transplants, and surgical procedures are all permitted.

- Prior to death, a family member (or, if unavailable, any practicing Muslim) reads the Qur'an (Islamic scripture) and prays; an imam (Muslim clergy) may be requested by the patient or family, but is not required.

- Before death, patients must face Mecca, confess sins, and beg forgiveness in the presence of family (or, if unavailable, before a practicing Muslim).

- After death, family or a Muslim of the same gender should wash and prepare the body and place the body in a position facing Mecca; in some instances, if necessary, health care professional may do this, but they must wear gloves (be sure to check with family on this).

- Burial is performed as soon as possible after death (no embalming); all five steps of the burial procedure must be followed (as above—washing, dressing, positioning, etc.).

- Cremation is not allowed.

- Autopsy is not allowed except for legal reasons; even in that case, no body part should be removed unless replaced with the body.

- Donation of body parts may not be allowed, although some permit organ or body donation (check with the family on specific beliefs).

- Organ transplantation to save a patient's life is often permitted.

- "Right to die" is not found in Islamic teachings; therefore, euthanasia or any shortening of life is not allowed; "do not resuscitate" (DNR) orders may not be permitted (check with the family).

• Death may be taboo subject for discussion and grief counselling seen as intrusive.

Miscellaneous Rituals/Customs

• Modesty is very important for women, who wear clothes that cover their entire body; this should be respected at all times during physical examination; they may not allow an internal prenatal exam.

• Gowns required for surgery and tests may be opposed; males are always covered from waist to knee.

• Women physicians and nurses are preferred for women; male physicians and nurses preferred for men; male staff should not examine women without their husbands or fathers present.

• Medical examination of either sex in front of groups of medical or nursing professionals is opposed.

• The husband needs to be present on admission since women are not allowed to sign consent forms or make decisions regarding family planning.

• Handshakes or any other contact between men and women is prohibited (except between husband and wife).

• Some Muslims may wear a black string on which words of Koran are attached; do not remove this and make efforts to keep it dry.

• Other jewelry, such as bangles, should not be removed unless necessary.

• Prayer is required five times a day (dawn, midday, midafternoon, sunset, and bedtime) and is done in private using a prayer rug, so accommodations should be made; washing is required before prayer (a bed-rest patient may require assistance).

• The Qur'an should not be touched by anyone who is not ritually clean.

• No objects should be placed on top of the Qur'an.

• Religious services are typically held on Friday.

• Three groups of Muslims: Sunni (traditionalists who follow Muhammad's way of teaching and living); Shiites (believe that only descendants of Muhammad should be spiritual leaders and that martyrdom is an honor); and Sufis (with mystical beliefs; monks and monasteries are common). Health rules may vary, so ask.

American Muslim Mission (Black Muslim)

Birth and Contraception

• No baptism practiced.

Diet

• Do not eat pork or traditional black American foods (corn bread, collard greens, etc.); alcohol and smoking are not permitted.

• May follow kosher diet.

Death, Dying, and Healing

• After death, family should be contacted before any care of patients is performed; special washing and shrouding of the body are required.

Miscellaneous Rituals/Customs

• A quiet time should be allowed for prayer.

• Black physicians are preferred for health care.

• Qur'an is holy scripture; five times daily prayer facing Mecca is practiced; buying on credit is not permitted; women wear head coverings.

EASTERN RELIGIOUS TRADITIONS

HINDUISM

Hinduism, the world's third largest religion (fourth largest in U.S.), has no specific founder or theological belief system, but consists of many different religious groups that have come about in India since about 1500 BC. Hindus recognize a single deity and view other gods or goddesses as manifestations of that one supreme God. However, it is pantheistic in its understanding of God; God or Brahman is seen as both one with the entire universe and simultaneously transcending it.

Birth and Contraception

• Hindus may prefer that education about family planning and obstetric services be performed by female physicians.

• Men are not usually present during birthing, although there is no rule against this.

• Hindus have many rituals and preferred foods during pregnancy to protect the fetus, so health professional should inquire about such factors.

• On the tenth or eleventh day, during a "cradle ceremony," babies are named and protected from evil spirits.

• Birth control, artificial insemination, amniocentesis, and genetic counseling are permitted.

Diet

• Often are vegetarians or partial vegetarians (accepting eggs, yogurt, milk, or cheese); usually refuse to eat meat and may refuse to eat any animal products.

• Dietary issues may influence medication regimens; thus, health professionals should ask about food rituals in relation to mealtimes and food selection practices.

• The right hand is used for eating and the left hand for toileting and personal hygiene (HPs need to be aware of this when illness affects the function of hands and arms).

Death, Dying, and Healing

• Blood products, drugs, vaccination, organ donation, and transplantation all allowed.

• Prefer to die at home close to the ground (mother earth) with incense burning.

• The environment around a dying person should be peaceful (as with Buddhism), since state of mind at death may affect the next life.

• After death, the priest performs a ceremony called *antyesti* to purify the deceased and console the bereaved; holy water is sprinkled on body and poured into the mouth of the deceased; thread may be tied around the neck or wrist, or a sacred basil leaf may be placed on the tongue.

• The body is usually cremated and ashes immersed or sprinkled in the holy rivers (when possible); until cremation, however, it is customary not to leave the body alone.

• The eldest son may say special prayers, and all male relatives may offer small balls of rice on behalf of the deceased.

• Women relatives may respond to the death with loud wailing, moaning, and beating their chests in front of the corpse; health care professionals should offer support and show respect for this aspect of Hindu culture.

• After death, Hindus believe in a transmigration of the soul or transfer of the soul into another body; bad deeds may result in someone being reborn in a worse life situation or even as an animal.

• Autopsy permitted; euthanasia not practiced.

Miscellaneous Rituals/Customs

• The father or husband is usually the spokesperson to whom questions should be directed.

• Personal hygiene is very important; bathing every day is necessary, but not after meals; hot water may be added to cold, but cold water not added to hot.

• There is a strong belief in karma, which involves the belief that the total compilation of all a person's past lives and actions result in the person's present condition, including his or her health or illness.

• Suffering (that may be seen as a result of one's deeds in past lives, i.e., karma) may compensate for bad deeds, so, for that reason, some Hindus may choose to suffer rather than seek medical care; future life after rebirth may depend on how illness, disability, and death are faced; this belief may affect compliance and medical decisions.

• Prayer for health is not emphasized; stoicism is encouraged.

• Ayurvedic medicines, based on traditional Indian medicine, are made from herbs or mixtures of herbs, either alone or in combination with minerals, metals, and other ingredients of animal origin, and may be taken along with allopathic medications or instead of them.

• Ayurvedic medicine believes that sickness results from an imbalance in Vata (wind), Pitta (bile), and Kapha (mucus); ayurvedic healers assist in returning the balance of Vata, Pitta, and Kapha in the body, resulting in cure of illness.

• Hindus may believe in and practice ayurvedic medicine and, since treatments may conflict or interact with allopathic treatments, health professionals need to know about this.

• Even among highly educated Hindus, the influence of supernatural forces and human excesses are considered important causes of illness (for example, excessive consumption of sweets causing round worms, too much sexual activity causing tuberculosis, improper eating habits cause diarrhea and cholera); this may interfere with prescribed medical or nursing treatments.

• Yoga is a Hindu health practice that about 5 percent of Americans are involved in that may increase strength, flexibility, and balance; transcendental meditation is a form of Hindu prayer that may help practitioners to relax and reduce stress.

• An extremely comprehensive article on Hindu belief, culture, and health practices has been written by Jayalakshmi Jambunathan, and should be referred to if more information is needed.[6]

BUDDHISM

Buddhism is the fourth largest religion in the world and the third largest religion in the United States, with over 1.5 million adherents. Buddhism emerged out of Hinduism, and has many similar practices.

Birth and Contraception

• Birth control, artificial insemination, and sterility testing are permitted.

• Abortion not permitted, since conception occurs when consciousness enters a fertilized egg and is considered the beginning of life;[7] however, circumstances of the patient may permit it.

• A ritual blessing of the baby is performed after birth, with giving of the dharma name.

• No official position on contraception.

Diet

• Depends on branch within Buddhism; some are vegetarians and others are non-vegetarians.

• Dietary restrictions may be strict in some branches, so health professionals should always ask.

• The traditional Buddhist healer may place the sick person on a strict diet of certain kinds of food, so the health professional should ask about this.

Death, Dying, and Healing

• Because of belief in reincarnation, death is the transition point for the next life.

• Pre-death counseling and rituals are important.

• A Buddhist representative should be notified in advance of death to ensure that the appropriate person is present to watch over dying person.

• It is extremely important to provide as much peace and quiet as possible for the dying person, since state of mind at the moment of death is believed to affect the quality of the next life (rebirth).

• Prayers are said and some times a special text is read to the person who is dying.

• After death, the consciousness of the person is felt to enter an intermediary body, called *bardo*, where it may remain for up to forty-nine days before being a new life.

• After death, the body must be kept in a peaceful state for three days and not touched or disturbed if possible.

• Extensive prayers are said to help the person's consciousness let go of the body and all of its attachments so that it can move into its next life, since this may help enhance the next rebirth.

• Family members may also meditate on the truth of impermanence—that nothing is permanent, but rather part of the cycle of birth, death, and rebirth until nirvana is achieved (for some).

- For the sick person, a Buddhist elder may follow a ritual of praying to the spirits of the patient's different body parts, promising to reward the spirits with rice wine and chicken; these may be given to the patient when healed to feed any returning spirits that may cause a relapse into illness.
- Will accept pain medications if in great discomfort as long as consciousness is not affected; clarity of mind, however, should be maintained.
- No restrictions to transplantation, organ donation, or autopsy (other than those listed above concerning treatment of body).
- Cremation is common.

Miscellaneous Rituals/Customs

- Illness may be viewed as a result of karma and a consequence of either a previous life or the present life (and this may influence whether health care is sought); not viewed as punishment from the Divine.
- No belief in "faith" healing.
- Some Buddhists wear Buddhas as necklace chains, which may be used for protection against evil spirits; the wearer must follow strict rules, and if these rules are broken, then this is believed to lead to nightmares, mental or physical illness, dangerous life situations, or result in the necklace losing its power.[8]
- Health professionals should ask about any chains or other jewelry that may have religious significance.
- Buddhists may believe that illness results from doing something offensive to deceased ancestors; for example, birth defects or chronic illnesses in babies may be viewed as resulting from sins committed by the baby or his/her parents in a past life.
- Traditional Buddhist medicine is practiced by a "medicine

man," who may use medicines made from herbs, roots or animal products, applying them to wounds or to the surrounding skin, giving them to be taken orally, encouraging the sick person to inhale the medicine through the mouth or nose, or administering it through a shower, bath, or sauna.

TAOISM

Taoism, Buddhism, and Confucianism are considered the three great religions of China. Today, Taoism has at least 20 million followers (most in Taiwan, but about 30,000 in North America), and many aspects of traditional Chinese medicine based on Taoism are becoming increasingly popular in the United States, especially as part of complementary and alternative medicine. The Tao is believed to be the cause of the universe and the force that flows through all life. The yin is considered the dark side and the yang is the light side. The yin-yang symbol (circle with teardrops inside that complement each other) represents the need to balance opposites in the universe, so that when the yin and yang are equally present, then all is calm and health is present. Traditional Chinese medicine emphasizes the body's *chi* or intrinsic energy, and disease is believed to result from the blocking of the chi or energy flow in the body.[9]

Birth and Contraception

• Chinese women prefer to receive care from female health professionals, especially with regard to gynecological, obstetrical, and prenatal care.

• Traditional Chinese medicine drugs/herbs and other treatments may be used for the unpleasant side-effects of pregnancy (nausea, etc.), so health professionals should ask about these.

- For the first month after birth, some Chinese women practice *Zuo yuezi*; this involves not only being off from work and staying at home, but also certain dietary practices.

- After birth, the mother may avoid "cold" foods (cereals, rice, wheat, potatoes, chickpeas, cold drinks, fruits, white sugar, milk, most vegetables and soy products) and prefer "hot" foods (pork, chicken, organ meats, eggs, brown sugar, ginger, nuts, honey, onions, tea, and coffee) to reachieve a balance of yin and yang in the body.

- Besides dietary changes, the first month after delivery is characterized by avoidance of physical work or any excessively pleasurable activities.

- Bathing (especially washing the hair) may be limited, and special "hot" types of bathing substances preferred.

- Contraception is allowed but should be discussed in private, away from other family members.

Diet

- Seek to achieve a balance of "hot" and "cold" foods to balance the yin and the yang (see above).

Death, Dying, and Healing

- End-of-life care and medical care in general may be influenced by Chinese patients' (and family members') unwillingness to complain of pain or other symptoms.

- Treatments for pain may be hampered by excessive fears of addiction, desire not to "bother" the doctor, or fatalistic beliefs related to suffering.

- Patients may show a reluctance to discuss a diagnosis, since in Eastern culture, families often withhold information from patients (particularly if the prognosis is bad).

• After death, the family is expected to prepare the body for burial (washing and dressing of body).

• Burial is preferred.

• No contraindications to receiving or giving organ transplants or receiving blood transfusions.

Miscellaneous Rituals/Customs

• Blockage of the *chi* or energy may be treated with acupuncture or use of herbal preparations or even heavy metals; health professionals should note that heavy metals lead to toxicity, particularly lead and mercury poisoning.

• In Taoism, there is no personal God to pray to, although Tao priests and some laypersons may seek solutions and greater awareness through meditation.

• Nevertheless, many of the common people believe in a myriad of spirits that exist throughout nature, worship different gods in heaven, and practice rituals to protect themselves from evil demons and ghosts.

OTHER RELIGIOUS TRADITIONS

NATIVE AMERICAN SPIRITUALITY

There are many different tribes with beliefs and rituals that differ greatly from each other (Inuit tribes in Alaska, as well as tribes in the eastern sub-Arctic, eastern woodlands, plains, and southwest United States).[10] Many Native Americans today are Christian and have been so for generations. Among non-Christian Native Americans, there is a common belief in a Creator, although many also believe in a mythical hero who is divine in nature. Lakota and Dakota Indians believe in a single spiritual force, the Wakan-Tanka. Several tribes have special prophets, such as Handsome

Lake among the Iroquois, Sweet Medicine among the Cheyenne, and White Buffalo Woman among the Lakota and Dakota tribes. Belief in spirits is also common, including those that control the weather, interact with people, or come from the underworld. There are many different beliefs about the afterlife; some may believe that we are reincarnated; that we return as ghosts; that there is an afterlife; or they may be uncertain. Often, people hold a combination of these beliefs.

Shamans and traditional medicine men (or women) are important healers in some traditions. Religious ceremonies are a central aspect of traditional Native American medicine. Some Native Americans may attend a "sweat lodge" for spiritual purification or healing of a disease. Healing methods may include the use of plant medicines and special ceremonies, dances, and chanting by the medicine man. Health care professionals should inquire about and accommodate these traditions.

Birth and Contraception

• Traditions vary by tribe.

• Birth may be followed by a ceremony with prayer (but this varies).

Diet

• Foods may be provided by family; ask patient/family about this.

Death, Dying, and Healing

• Burning of sacred plants (sage, cedar, osha root, copal, pine, juniper) may be an important ritual for some tribes when a member is sick.

• The body may be prepared for burial by family or members of tribe (ask about this).

• After death, some families/tribes may not touch the person's clothes or belongings (ask about this).

• Rituals and ceremonies are common after death to facilitate guiding the deceased person's spirit to the supernatural world.

Miscellaneous Rituals/Customs

• Illness is thought to be caused by being out of balance with nature and the environment.

• Ceremonies with prayer/chanting and smudging may be used to return physical, emotional, and spiritual balance and harmony.

• Hospital environments may need to be altered to allow this ceremonial burning (smudging), or arrangements made so that this can be done safely in a para-hospital environment; this is very important for some Native Americans and, if not allowed, can create conflict.

• A medicine bag may be worn around the neck, and religious articles and other sacred objects may be worn on the body or clothes; always ask permission before touching or removing.

• Ask if the patient would like to include or contact an elder, medicine person, or spiritual leader (may not be called clergy) to assist with healing.

FOLK RELIGIONS

In addition to the major religious traditions discussed above, there are also many folk religions around the world and among immigrants who come to the United States. If requested, practitioners from these traditions may be invited to assist with sick patients.

Patients may not talk about these beliefs unless specifically asked.

Santeria is a religion of Caribbean origin, with elements of Roman Catholicism mixed in. There is belief in a supreme deity and a lesser deity. Ritual sacrifices and possession states are important aspects of ceremonies for healing.[11]

Curanderisimo is a Latino or Hispanic folk religion that includes a classification of illness such as "evil eye," "fright," "blockage," and "fallen fontanelle." One study found that 32–96 percent of Mexican American households treated members for Hispanic folk illnesses.[12] Curanderos (men) or curanderas (women) are folk healers who practice a combination of shamanic, herbal, and first-aid types of healing.

Vodun (or voodoo) is common among Haitians or others from the West Indies. Voodoo rituals are very important for healing, and patients may request a voodoo priest to carry out rituals for healing and protection.[13]

NEW AGE SPIRITUALITY

Approximately 20 percent of the U.S. population indicates that they are spiritual but not religious, and many of these persons (but certainly not all) may be involved in New Age spiritual practices. New Age believers may have a variety of paranormal beliefs that could affect health care, and they often have great interest in Eastern religious healing methods such as transcendental meditation (Hindu), mindfulness meditation (Buddhist), "therapeutic touch" (redistributes healing energy that in Chinese religions is called *chi*), Reiki (Japanese type of healing), or Prana (life form or breath, important in yoga).

Health professionals should provide a quiet time and space to allow these practices if the patient desires. New Age believers may request alternative practitioners proficient in the above techniques to assist in care, and this should be permitted (as long as it doesn't substantially interfere with allopathic medical treatments).

NO AFFILIATION

Health professionals should never assume that patients without a religious affiliation (11% of the population) have no spiritual beliefs or practices that could influence their health care. Since these patients are not affiliated with any religious tradition or community, the chaplain may be the only person in the medical setting who can meet their spiritual needs (since they will not have community clergy). Of course, those without a religious affiliation may also wish to avoid inquiry into these aspects of their lives, and this should always be respected.

SUMMARY AND CONCLUSION

The information presented above represents a brief and incomplete synopsis of the health care practices of a number of major religious traditions that HPs are likely to encounter in clinical practice. It is important to bear in mind, however, that patients may or may not adhere to the health care practices of their religious tradition, and health care practices may vary widely within branches of a particular faith tradition, so it is always important to check with the patient and family regarding the religious practices related to health and health care that are important to them.

CHAPTER 14

SUMMARY OF KEY POINTS

R egardless of whether the reader is a physician, nurse, social worker, psychologist, counselor, rehabilitation specialist, or other allied health professional, there are certain key points that should be thoroughly understood after completing this book.[1] If these points are followed and integrated into clinical practice, then HPs will understand why addressing spiritual aspects is essential for whole-person health care, spiritual needs of patients will be recognized and appropriately addressed, and patients will be protected from the coercion and confusion that results when HPs overstep the bounds of their expertise. Furthermore, HPs will avoid duplicating each other's efforts and stepping on each other's toes, and communication and cooperation about these issues will be maximized.

1. There are reasons why HPs should communicate with patients about religious or spiritual issues:

• Many patients are religious, have spiritual needs, wish HPs to know about those beliefs, and often want them addressed as part of their health care.

• Religion can influence patients' ability to cope with illness, and HPs who care for them should be aware of this.

• Most patients in health care settings are isolated from their religious communities and from experts capable of specifically addressing spiritual needs related to their illnesses and hospital environment.

• Religious beliefs (and health practices related to religious traditions) can directly impact how patients wish to be cared for, may impact medical decisions, and at times may conflict with medical treatments.

• There is a growing volume of research indicating that religious involvement, in general, is associated with mental and physical health, and likely affects health outcomes in one way or another.

• Religion influences the support and care that patients receive in the community where they live, and this can affect whether or not they receive medical care and are compliant with medical treatments.

2. To learn about patients' religious/spirituality beliefs and traditions (or lack thereof), HPs should take a brief spiritual history on all seriously or chronically ill patients admitted to the hospital or other health care settings, and on new patients being seen for the first time; in this way, HPs will become aware of beliefs or practices that affect health care and can identify spiritual needs.

3. HPs (non-chaplains) should be responsible for "screening" patients for spiritual needs and identifying potential spiritual conflicts with the medical care plan since, given current resources, only one in five patients is likely to see a chaplain.

4. Information learned from the spiritual history should be documented in a special place in the medical record so that other HPs do not repeat the screening spiritual history; the spiritual assessment conducted by the chaplain and any follow-up visits and progress should likewise be documented here.

5. The physician, as head of the health care team, should conduct the screening spiritual history; if he or she fails to do so, then the responsibility falls on the nurse; if the nurse fails to do so, then the responsibility falls to the social worker, counselor, or other allied health professional who regularly sees the patient (occupational or physical therapy). A routine procedure should be established in this regard.

6. The religious or spiritual beliefs of patients should be respected and attempts made to understand them without judgment. If the HP is knowledgeable about the beliefs and they do not appear to be outright harmful, then supporting and accommodating a patient's beliefs and religious practices is appropriate.

7. If an HP identifies spiritual needs or conflicts, is not familiar with the patient's religious beliefs, or suspects that such beliefs may be harmful, then the HP should always refer (with the patient's consent) to professional health care chaplains, who have the time and expertise to deal with these issues; if the patient refuses referral, then the HP should still consult with a chaplain for guidance and direction on how he or she should handle the situation.

8. HPs should know the qualifications of chaplains working in their area and find out how chaplains can help in addressing the spiritual needs of patients, in dealing with sticky ethical issues, and in working with patients, families, and staff who are struggling with emotional problems related to illness and loss; the health care chaplain should be included as a regular member of the multidisciplinary health care team and spiritual care plans should

always be developed either by or in consultation with the chaplain.

9. Most of the time, HPs without clinical pastoral education should not attempt to address spiritual needs or provide advice about spiritual matters to patients since this is not in their area of expertise and will take time away from the services that they are trained to deliver.

10. The screening spiritual history and any interventions (prayer, chaplain referral) must always be patient centered and patient desired; the patient must have the free and uncoerced freedom of choice, including the choice not to be asked questions about spiritual matters or engage in spiritual activities with HPs (including chaplains).

11. HPs should not ask patients to pray with them (initiate prayer); however, HPs may inform religious patients that they will pray with patients if that is desired, and then leave it up to the patient to *later* initiate the request (to ensure that the choice is completely free and uncoerced). Prayer with patients should be done quietly and privately, and care taken to ensure that it does not disturb other patients.

12. HPs, especially mental health care providers, should be aware of boundary issues. HPs should never seek to change the religious beliefs of patients (either evangelize them, or discourage religious involvement); if there is any reason to believe that religious beliefs/activities are harmful or interfering with patient care, consult with a professional chaplain.

13. The religious beliefs of HPs (or lack thereof) should not influence whether they take a spiritual history, show respect and value for patients' beliefs, or refer patients to chaplains (since these are patient-centered activities, not HP centered). HP discomfort over discussing such issues must be overcome by training and practice.

14. HPs should learn about the health-related religious tradi-

tions of the patients they are most likely to encounter, or know where to find this information if needed.

15. If spiritual needs are uncovered and a patient is referred to the chaplain, the HP should follow up later to see if the patient's spiritual needs were adequately addressed (given their potential impact on health and health outcomes). At the time of discharge, the HP (often a social worker), together with the chaplain, should develop a spiritual care discharge plan to ensure that continuity of spiritual care is maintained between hospital and community or other institution.

16. HPs should never argue with patients about religious matters, even if they conflict with medical care, but rather seek to understand them and convey respect; again, pastoral care experts should be consulted on how to proceed if there is any potential for conflict.

CONCLUSION

In today's health care system, it is tempting for clinicians to simply become technicians and focus on the pressing physical health issues at hand. Of course, this is our primary responsibility and must be done rigorously and competently. Meeting only the physical needs of patients, however, is not worth the amount of effort, time, and emotional energy involved in this line of work, and we will miss out on the professional satisfaction that comes from treating the whole person. In the past, there was much more to being a health professional than just the technical aspects, and if we are to avoid becoming burned out in the future, we must be much more than just technicians. Addressing spiritual issues in clinical practice can bring life back into our profession and, for many of our patients, can help them regain their lives by finding hope, meaning, and healing.

NOTES

INTRODUCTION

1. H. G. Koenig, M. McCullough, and D. B. Larson, *Handbook of Religion and Health* (New York: Oxford University Press, 2001).

2. H. G. Koenig, "Religion, Spirituality and Health: Understanding the Mechanisms," in *Spiritual Dimensions of Nursing*, 2nd ed., ed. V. B. Carson and H. G. Koenig (not yet published).

3. Joint Commission for the Accreditation of Hospital Organizations, http://www.jointcommission.org/AccreditationPrograms/Hospitals/Standards/FAQs/Provision+of+Care/Assessment/Spiritual_Assessment.htm (last revised January 1, 2004).

4. B. J. Kozier, G. Erb, A. J. Berman, and S. Snyder, *Fundamentals of Nursing: Concepts, Process, and Practice*, 7th ed. (Englewood Cliffs, NJ: Prentice Hall, 2003).

5. NANDA International, *Nursing Diagnoses: Definitions and Classifications 2007–2008* (St. Louis, MO: Elsevier, 2006).

6. J. M. Dochterman and G. M. Bulechek, *Nursing Interventions Classification (NIC)*, 4th ed. (St. Louis, MO: Mosby, 2003).

7. S. Moorhead, M. Johnson, and M. L. Maas, *Nursing Outcome Classification (NOC)*, 3rd ed. (St. Louis, MO: Mosby, 2003).

8. Association of American Medical Colleges, "Contemporary Issues in Medicine: Communication in Medicine," Medical School Objectives Project, Report III, 1999, http://www.aamc.org/meded/msop/msop3.pdf, p. 25.

9. C. M. Puchalski, "Spirituality and Medicine: Curricula in Medical Education," *Journal of Cancer Education* 21, no. 1 (2006): 14–18; *John Templeton Foundation Capabilities Report* (West Conshohocken, PA: Templeton Foundation, 2006), 68.

10. J. T. Chibnall and C. A. Brooks, "Religion in the Clinic: The Role of Physician Beliefs," *Southern Medical Journal* 94 (2001): 374–79; F. A. Curlin, M. H. Chin, S. A. Sellergren, C. J. Roach, and J. D. Lantos, "The Association of Physicians' Religious Characteristics with Their Attitudes and Self-Reported Behaviors Regarding Religion and Spirituality in the Clinical Encounter," *Medical Care* 44 (2006): 446–53.

11. D. E. King and B. J. Wells, "End-of-Life Issues and Spiritual Histories," *Southern Medical Journal* 96 (2003): 391–93.

12. D. J. Hufford, "An Analysis of the Field of Spirituality, Religion, and Health," Area 1 Field Analysis, 2005, www.metanexus.net/tarp, p. 23.

13. Joint Commission for the Accreditation of Hospital Organizations, http://www.jointcommission.org/AccreditationPrograms/Hospitals/Standards/FAQs/Provision+of+Care/Assessment/Spiritual_Assessment.htm (last revised January 1, 2004).

14. G. Fitchett, L. A. Burton, and A. B. Sivan, "The Religious Needs and Resources of Psychiatric Patients," *Journal of Nervous and Mental Disease* 185 (1997): 320–26.

15. L. VandeCreek and B. Cooke, "Hospital Pastoral Care Practices of Parish Clergy," *Research in the Social Scientific Study of Religion* 7 (1996): 253–64.

16. L. VandeCreek, "How Has Health Care Reform Affected Professional Chaplaincy Programs and How Are Department Directors Responding?" *Journal of Health Care Chaplaincy* 10, no. 1 (2000): 7–17.

17. J. Bailey, "Legislature Approves Budget Cuts: Cuts Also Endanger Central State Chaplaincy Program," *The Union-Recorder* (Milledgeville, GA), August 29, 1991, 1; Association of Mental Health Clergy, "Here We Are Again! Crisis in Georgia," *AMHC Newsletter* 3, no. 10 (September 1991): 1.

18. K. J. Flannelly, K. Galek, and G. F. Handzo, "To What Extent Are the Spiritual Needs of Hospital Patients Being Met?" *International Journal of Psychiatry in Medicine* 35, no. 3 (2005): 319–23.

19. G. Handzo and H. G. Koenig, "Spiritual Care: Whose Job Is It Anyway?" *Southern Medical Journal* 97 (2004): 1242–44.

20. P. A. Clark, M. Drain, and M. P. Malone, "Addressing Patients' Emotional and Spiritual Needs," *Joint Commission Journal on Quality and Safety* 29 (2003): 659–70.

21. C. May and N. Mead, "Patient-Centeredness: A History," in *General Practice and Ethics Uncertainty and Responsibility*, ed. C. Dowrick and I. Firth (London: Routledge, 1999), 76–90.

22. L. B. Carey, C. J. Newell, and B. Rumbold, "Pain Control and Chaplaincy in Australia," *Journal of Pain and Symptom Management* 32, no. 6 (2006): 589-600.

CHAPTER 1:*WHY* INCLUDE SPIRITUALITY?

1. Princeton Religion Research Center, *Religion in America* (Princeton, NJ: The Gallup Poll, 1996).

2. F. Newport, "Religion Most Important to Blacks, Women, and Older Americans," *The Gallup Brain*, 2006, http://brain.gallup.com/content/default. aspx?ci=25585.

3. R. C. Fuller, *Spiritual but Not Religious* (New York: Oxford University Press, 2005).

4. H. G. Koenig, L. K. George, and P. Titus, "Religion, Spirituality and Health in Medically Ill Hospitalized Older Patients," *Journal of the American Geriatrics Association* 52 (2004): 554–62.

5. G. Fitchett, L. A. Burton, and A. B. Sivan, "The Religious Needs and Resources of Psychiatric Patients," *Journal of Nervous and Mental Disease* 185 (1997): 320–26.

6. D. E. King and B. Bushwick, "Beliefs and Attitudes of Hospital Inpatients about Faith Healing and Prayer," *Journal of Family Practice* 39 (1994): 349–52.

7. C. D. MacLean, B. Susi, N. Phifer, L. Schultz, D. Bynum, M. Franco, A. Klioze, M. Monroe, J. Garrett, and S. Cykert, "Patient Preference for Physician Discussion and Practice of Spirituality," *Journal of General Internal Medicine* 18 (2003): 38–43; King and Bushwick, "Beliefs and Attitudes of Hospital Inpatients about Faith Healing and Prayer"; T. P. Daaleman and D. E. Nease, "Patient Attitudes Regarding Physician Inquiry into Spiritual and Religious Issues," *Journal of Family Practice* 39 (1994): 564–68; T. A. Maugans and W. C. Wadland, "Religion and Family Medicine: A Survey of Physicians and Patients," *Journal of Family Practice* 32 (1991): 210–13; B. E. Miller, B. Pittman, and C. Strong, "Gynecologic Cancer Patients' Psychosocial Needs and Their Views on the Physician's Role in Meeting Those Needs," *International Journal of Gynecological Cancer* 13, no. 2 (2003): 111–19; O. Oyama and H. G. Koenig, "Religious Beliefs and Practices in Family Medicine," *Archives of Family Medicine* 7 (1998): 431–35; J. L. Hamilton and J. P. Levine, "Neo-Pagan Patients' Preferences Regarding Physician Discussion of Spirituality," *Family Medicine* 38, no. 2 (2006): 83–84.

8. Oyama and Koenig, "Religious Beliefs and Practices in Family Medicine."

9. L. C. Kaldjian, J. F. Jekel, and G. Friedland, "End-of-Life Decisions in HIV-Positive Patients: The Role of Spiritual Beliefs," *AIDS* 12, no. 1 (1998): 103–7.

10. T. McNichol, "The New Faith in Medicine," *USA Weekend*, April 5–7, 1996, 5.

11. J. Ehman, B. Ott, T. Short, R. Ciampa, and J. Hansen-Flaschen, "Do Patients Want Physicians to Inquire about Their Spiritual or Religious Beliefs if They Become Gravely Ill?" *Archives of Internal Medicine* 159 (1999): 1803–6;

Hamilton and Levine, "Neo-Pagan Patients' Preferences Regarding Physician Discussion of Spirituality."

12. J. L. Kristeller, M. Rhodes, L. D. Cripe, and V. Sheets, "Oncologist Assisted Spiritual Intervention Study (OASIS): Patient Acceptability and Initial Evidence of Effects," *International Journal of Psychiatry in Medicine* 35 (2005): 329–47.

13. Ehman et al., "Do Patients Want Physicians to Inquire about Their Spiritual or Religious Beliefs if They Become Gravely Ill?"; Hamilton and Levine, "Neo-Pagan Patients' Preferences Regarding Physician Discussion of Spirituality."

14. MacLean et al., "Patient Preference for Physician Discussion"; King and Bushwick, "Beliefs and Attitudes of Hospital Inpatients about Faith Healing and Prayer"; Oyama and Koenig, "Religious Beliefs and Practices in Family Medicine"; Hamilton and Levine, "Neo-Pagan Patients' Preferences Regarding Physician Discussion of Spirituality"; H. G. Koenig, M. Smiley, and J. Gonzales, *Religion, Health, and Aging* (Westport, CT: Greenwood Press, 1988).

15. Kaldjian, Jekel, and Friedland, "End-of-Life Decisions in HIV-Positive Patients: The Role of Spiritual Beliefs."

16. McNichol, "The New Faith in Medicine"; Ehman et al., "Do Patients Want Physicians to Inquire about Their Spiritual or Religious Beliefs if They Become Gravely Ill?"; King and Bushwick, "Beliefs and Attitudes of Hospital Inpatients about Faith Healing and Prayer."

17. C. J. Mansfield, J. Mitchell, and D. E. King, "The Doctor as God's Mechanic? Beliefs in the Southeastern United States," *Social Science & Medicine* 54, no. 3 (2002): 399–409.

18. MacLean et al., "Patient Preference for Physician Discussion."

19. Princeton Religion Research Center, *Religion in America.*

20. M. A. Schuster, B. D. Stein, L. H. Jaycox, R. L. Collins, G. N. Marshall, M. N. Elliott, A. J. Zhou, D. E. Kanouse, J. L. Morrison, and S. H. Berry, "A National Survey of Stress Reactions after the September 11, 2001, Terrorist Attacks," *New England Journal of Medicine* 345 (2001): 1507–12.

21. H. G. Koenig, "Religious Beliefs and Practices of Hospitalized Medically Ill Older Adults," *International Journal of Geriatric Psychiatry* 13 (1998): 213–24.

22. T. L. Saudia, M. R. Kinney, K. C. Brown, and L. Young-Ward, "Health Locus of Control and Helpfulness of Prayer," *Heart and Lung* 20 (1991): 60–65.

23. T. A. Cronan, R. M. Kaplan, L. Posner, E. Lumberg, and F. Kozin, "Prevalence of the Use of Unconventional Remedies for Arthritis in a Metropolitan Community," *Arthritis and Rheumatism* 32 (1989): 1604–7.

24. A. P. Tix and P. A. Frazier, "The Use of Religious Coping During Stressful Life Events: Main Effects, Moderation, and Mediation," *Journal of Consulting and Clinical Psychology* 66 (1997): 411–22.

25. R. C. Stern, E. R. Canda, and C. F. Doershuk, "Use of Nonmedical

Treatment by Cystic Fibrosis Patients," *Journal of Adolescent Health* 13 (1992): 612–15.

26. Ibid.

27. K. O. Ell, J. E. Mantell, M. B. Hamovitch, and R. H. Nishimoto, "Social Support, Sense of Control, and Coping among Patients with Breast, Lung, or Colorectal Cancer," *Journal of Psychosocial Oncology* 7 (1989): 63–89.

28. J. A. Roberts, D. Brown, T. Elkins, and D. B. Larson, "Factors Influencing Views of Patients with Gynecologic Cancer about End-of-Life Decisions," *American Journal of Obstetrics and Gynecology* 176 (1997): 166–72.

29. R. A. Jenkins, "Religion and HIV: Implications for Research and Intervention," *Journal of Social Issues* (1995): 131–44.

30. A. F. Abraido-Lanza, C. Guier, and T. A. Revenson, "Coping and Social Support Resources among Latinas with Arthritis," *Arthritis Care and Research* 9, no. 6 (1996): 501–8.

31. T. J. Silber and M. Reilly, "Spiritual and Religious Concerns of the Hospitalized Adolescent," *Adolescence* 20 (1985): 217–24.

32. H. G. Koenig, D. K. Weiner, B. L. Peterson, K. G. Meador, and F. J. Keefe, "Religious Coping in Institutionalized Elderly Patients," *International Journal of Psychiatry in Medicine* 27 (1998): 365–76.

33. S. D. Wright, C. C. Pratt, and V. L. Schmall, "Spiritual Support for Caregivers of Dementia Patients," *Journal of Religion and Health* 24 (1985): 31–38.

34. The privacy rule of the Health Insurance Portability and Accountability Act prevents any protected health information (including a patient's identify) to be released by a hospital without the explicit consent of the patient.

35. Ehman et al., "Do Patients Want Physicians to Inquire about Their Spiritual or Religious Beliefs if They Become Gravely Ill?"

36. Hamilton and Levine, "Neo-Pagan Patients' Preferences Regarding Physician Discussion of Spirituality."

37. Kaldjian, Jekel, and Friedland, "End-of-Life Decisions in HIV-Positive Patients: The Role of Spiritual Beliefs."

38. G. A. Silvestri, S. Knittig, J. S. Zoller, et al., "Importance of Faith on Medical Decisions Regarding Cancer Care," *Journal of Clinical Oncology* 21 (2003): 1379–82.

39. H. G. Koenig, M. McCullough, and D. B. Larson, *Handbook of Religion and Health* (New York: Oxford University Press, 2001).

40. H. G. Koenig, "An 83-Year-Old Woman with Chronic Illness and Strong Religious Beliefs," *Journal of the American Medical Association* 288, no. 4 (2002): 487–93.

41. H. G. Koenig, H. J. Cohen, D. G. Blazer, C. Pieper, K. G. Meador, F. Shelp, V. Goli, and R. DiPasquale, "Religious Coping and Depression in Elderly Hospitalized Medically Ill Men," *American Journal of Psychiatry* 149 (1992): 1693–1700; H. G. Koenig, "Religion and Depression in Older Medical

Inpatients," *American Journal of Geriatric Psychiatry* 15 (2007):000-000 (April), in press; P. Pressman, J. S. Lyons, D. B. Larson, and J. J. Strain, "Religious Belief, Depression, and Ambulation Status in Elderly Women with Broken Hips," *American Journal of Psychiatry* 147 (1990): 758–59.

42. H. G. Koenig, L. K. George, and B. L. Peterson, "Religiosity and Remission from Depression in Medically Ill Older Patients," *American Journal of Psychiatry* 155 (1998): 536–42; H. G. Koenig, "Religion and Remission of Depression in Medical Inpatients with Heart Failure/Pulmonary Disease," *Journal of Nervous and Mental Disease* 195 (2007): (May), in press.

43. P. V. Rabins, M. D. Fitting, J. Eastham, and J. Zabora, "Emotional Adaptation over Time in Care-givers for Chronically Ill Elderly People," *Age and Ageing* 19 (1990): 185–90.

44. Koenig, McCullough, and Larson, *Handbook of Religion and Health.*

45. Ibid.

46. S. Freud, "Civilization and Its Discontents," in *Standard Edition of the Complete Psychological Works of Sigmund Freud,* ed. and trans. J. Strachey (1930; London: Hogarth Press, 1962), 25.

47. Koenig, McCullough, and Larson, *Handbook of Religion and Health.*

48. C. G. Ellison and L. K. George, "Religious Involvement, Social Ties, and Social Support in a Southeastern Community," *Journal for the Scientific Study of Religion* 33 (1994): 46–61.

49. B. S. McEwen, "Protective and Damaging Effects of Stress Mediators," *New England Journal of Medicine* 338 (1998): 171–79.

50. E. S. Epel, E. H. Blackburn, J. Lin, F. S. Dhabhar, N. E. Adler, J. D. Morrow, and R. M. Cawthon, "Accelerated Telomere Shortening in Response to Life Stress," *Proceedings of the National Academy of Sciences of the United States of America* 101, no. 49 (2004): 17312–15.

51. H. G. Koenig, H. J. Cohen, L. K. George, J. C. Hays, D. B. Larson, and D. G. Blazer, "Attendance at Religious Services, Interleukin-6, and Other Biological Indicators of Immune Function in Older Adults," *International Journal of Psychiatry in Medicine* 27 (1997): 233–50.

52. S. K. Lutgendorf, D. Russell, P. Ullrich, T. B. Harris, and R. Wallace, "Religious Participation, Interleukin-6, and Mortality in Older Adults," *Health Psychology* 23, no. 5 (2004): 465–75.

53. S. E. Sephton, C. Koopman, M. Schaal, C. Thoreson, and D. Spiegel, "Spiritual Expression and Immune Status in Women with Metastatic Breast Cancer: An Exploratory Study," *Breast Journal* 7 (2001): 345–53.

54. T. E. Woods, M. H. Antoni, G. H. Ironson, and D. W. Kling, "Religiosity Is Associated with Affective and Immune Status in Symptomatic HIV-Infected Gay Men," *Journal of Psychosomatic Research* 46 (1999): 165–76.

55. G. Ironson, R. Stuetzie, and M. A. Fletcher, "An Increase in Religiousness/Spirituality Occurs after HIV Diagnosis and Predicts Slower Disease Progression over 4 Years in People with HIV," *Journal of General Internal Medicine* 21 (2006): S62–68.

56. G. Ironson, G. F. Solomon, E. G. Balbin, et al., "Spirituality and Religiousness Are Associated with Long Survival, Health Behaviors, Less Distress, and Lower Cortisol in People Living with HIV/AIDS: The IWORSHIP Scale, Its Validity and Reliability," *Annals of Behavioral Medicine* 24 (2002): 34–48.

57. E. A. Dedert, J. L. Studts, I. Weissbecker, P. G. Salmon, P. L. Banis, and S. E. Sephton, "Private Religious Practice: Protection of Cortisol Rhythms among Women with Fibromyalgia," *International Journal of Psychiatry in Medicine* 34 (2004): 61–77.

58. Koenig, McCullough, and Larson, *Handbook of Religion and Health*.

59. A. Colantonio, S. V. Kasl, and A. M. Ostfeld, "Depressive Symptoms and Other Psychosocial Factors as Predictors of Stroke in the Elderly," *American Journal of Epidemiology* 136 (1992): 884–94.

60. U. Goldbourt, S. Yaari, and J. H. Medalie, "Factors Predictive of Long-Term Coronary Heart Disease Mortality among 10,059 Male Israeli Civil Servants and Municipal Employees," *Cardiology* 82 (1993): 100–121.

61. Koenig, McCullough, and Larson, *Handbook of Religion and Health*.

62. M. E. McCullough, W. T. Hoyt, D. B. Larson, H. G. Koenig, and C. Thoresen, "Religious Involvement and Mortality: A Meta-Analytic Review," *Health Psychology* 19 (2000): 211–22.

63. R. Hummer, R. Rogers, C. Nam, and C. G. Ellison, "Religious Involvement and U.S. Adult Mortality," *Demography* 36 (1999): 273–85.

64. H. G. Koenig, J. C. Hays, D. B. Larson, L. K. George, H. J. Cohen, M. McCullough, K. Meador, D. G. Blazer, "Does Religious Attendance Prolong Survival?: A Six-Year Follow-up Study of 3,968 Older Adults," *Journal of Gerontology, Medical Sciences* 54A (1999): M370–77; W. J. Strawbridge, S. J. Shema, R. D. Cohen, and G. A. Kaplan, "Religious Attendance Increases Survival by Improving and Maintaining Good Health Behaviors, Mental Health, and Social Relationships," *Annals of Behavioral Medicine* 23, no. 1 (2001): 68–74.

65. W. J. Strawbridge, R. D. Cohen, S. J. Shema, and G. A. Kaplan, "Frequent Attendance at Religious Services and Mortality over 28 Years," *American Journal of Public Health* 87 (1997): 957–61; H. G. Koenig, E. Idler, S. Kasl, J. Hays, L. K. George, M. Musick, D. B. Larson, T. Collins, and H. Benson, "Religion, Spirituality, and Medicine: A Rebuttal to Skeptics," *International Journal of Psychiatry in Medicine* 29 (1999): 123–31.

66. Lutgendorf et al., "Religious Participation, Interleukin-6, and Mortality in Older Adults"; Ironson, Stuetzie, and Flectcher, "An Increase in Religiousness/Spirituality Occurs after HIV Diagnosis and Predicts Slower Disease Progression over 4 Years in People with HIV."

67. E. L. Idler and S. V. Kasl, "Religion among Disabled and Nondisabled Elderly Persons, II: Attendance at Religious Services as a Predictor of the Course of Disability," *Journal of Gerontology* 52B (1997): 306–16; N. S. Park, D. L. Klemmack, L. L. Roff, M. W. Parker, and H. G. Koenig, "Religiousness and

Longitudinal Trajectories in Elders' Functional Status," (2007), submitted; C. A. Reyes-Ortiz, H. Ayele, T. Mulligan, D. V. Espino, I. M. Berges, and K. S. Markides, "Higher Church Attendance Predicts Lower Fear of Falling in Older Mexican-Americans," *Aging and Mental Health* 10, no. 1 (2006): 13–18.

68. T. Hill, A. Burdette, J. Angel, et al., "Religious Attendance and Cognitive Functioning among Older Mexican Americans," *Journal of Gerontology* 61 (2006): P3–9; P. Van Ness and S. Kasl, "Religion and Cognitive Dysfunction in an Elderly Cohort," *Journal of Gerontology* 58B (2003): S21–29.

69. Y. Kaufman, A. Binns, and M. Freedman, "The Effects of Spirituality and Religiosity on the Rates of Cognitive Decline and Quality of Life in Alzheimer's Disease," American Academy of Neurology, Miami, FL, 2005.

70. T. E. Oxman, D. H. Freeman, and E. D. Manheimer, "Lack of Social Participation or Religious Strength and Comfort as Risk Factors for Death after Cardiac Surgery in the Elderly," *Psychosomatic Medicine* 57 (1995): 5–15.

71. R. J. Contrada, T. M. Goyal, C. Cather, L. Rafalson, E. L. Idler, T. J. Krause, "Psychosocial Factors in Outcomes of Heart Surgery: The Impact of Religious Involvement and Depressive Symptoms," *Health Psychology* 23 (2004): 227–38.

72. K. I. Pargament, H. G. Koenig, N. Tarakeshwar, and J. Hahn, "Religious Struggle as a Predictor of Mortality among Medically Ill Elderly Patients: A Two-Year Longitudinal Study," *Archives of Internal Medicine* 161 (2001): 1881–85.

73. K. Nelson, A. M. Geiger, and C. M. Mangione, "Effect of Health Beliefs on Delays in Care for Abnormal Cervical Cytology in a Multiethnic Population," *Journal of General Internal Medicine* 17, no. 9 (2002): 709–16; L. R. Chavez, F. A. Hubbell, S. I. Mishra, and R. B. Valdez, "The Influence of Fatalism on Self-Reported Use of Papanicolaou Smears," *American Journal of Preventive Medicine* 13 (1997): 418–24; D. Cohen-Mor, *A Matter of Fate: The Concept of Fate in the Arab World as Reflected in Modern Arabic Literature* (New York: Oxford University Press, 2001); R. C. Soloman, "Freedom," in *Introducing Philosophy: A Text with Integrated Readings*, 8th ed. (New York: Oxford University Press, 2004), chap. 7, with section on fatalism and karma.

74. H. G. Koenig and D. B. Larson, "Use of Hospital Services, Church Attendance, and Religious Affiliation," *Southern Medical Journal* 91 (1998): 925–32.

75. H. G. Koenig, L. K. George, P. Titus, and K. G. Meador, "Religion, Spirituality, Acute Hospital and Long-Term Care Use by Older Patients," *Archives of Internal Medicine* 164 (2004): 1579–85.

76. S. Freud, "Future of an Illusion," in *Standard Edition of the Complete Psychological Works of Sigmund Freud*, ed. and trans. J. Strachey (1927; London: Hogarth Press, 1962), 43.

77. See JCAHO Web site, http://www.jointcommission.org/AccreditationPrograms/HomeCare/Standards/FAQs/Provision+of+Care/Assessment/Spiritual_Assessment.htm.

78. M. R. Ellis, D. C. Vinson, and B. Ewigman, "Addressing Spiritual Concerns of Patients: Family Physicians' Attitudes and Practices," *Journal of Family Practice* 48 (1999): 105–9.

79. M. H. Monroe, D. Bynum, B. Susi, N. Phifer, L. Schultz, M. Franco, C. D. MacLean, S. Cykert, and J. Garrett, "Primary Care Physicians Preferences Regarding Spiritual Behavior in Medical Practice," *Archives of Internal Medicine* 163 (2003): 2751–56.

80. T. A. Maugans and W. C. Wadland, "Religion and Family Medicine: A Survey of Physicians and Patients," *Journal of Family Practice* 32 (1991): 210–13.

81. F. A. Curlin, M. H. Chin, S. A. Sellergren, C. J. Roach, and J. D. Lantos, "The Association of Physicians' Religious Characteristics with Their Attitudes and Self-Reported Behaviors Regarding Religion and Spirituality in the Clinical Encounter," *Medical Care* 44 (2006): 446–53.

82. J. T. Chibnall and C. A. Brooks, "Religion in the Clinic: The Role of Physician Beliefs," *Southern Medical Journal* 94 (2001): 374–79; D. E. King and B. J. Wells, "End-of-Life Issues and Spiritual Histories," *Southern Medical Journal* 96 (2003): 391–93.

83. H. G. Koenig, L. Bearon, and R. Dayringer, "Physician Perspectives on the Role of Religion in the Physician–Older Patient Relationship," *Journal of Family Practice* 28 (1989): 441–48.

84. Monroe et al., *Archives of Internal Medicine.*

85. Curlin et al., "The Association of Physicians' Religious Characteristics with Their Attitudes and Self-Reported Behaviors Regarding Religion and Spirituality in the Clinical Encounter."

86. H. G. Koenig, M. E. McCollough, and D. B. Larson, "Historical Perspective," in *Handbook of Religion and Health,* chap. 2; H. G. Koenig, "History of Mental Health Care," in *Faith and Mental Health* (Philadelphia: Templeton Foundation Press, 2005), chap. 2.

CHAPTER 2: *HOW* TO INCLUDE SPIRITUALITY

1. A. Moreira-Almeida and H. G. Koenig, "Retaining the Meaning of the Words Religiousness And Spirituality: A Commentary on the WHOQOL SRPB Group's 'A Cross-Cultural Study of Spirituality, Religion, and Personal Beliefs as Components of Quality of Life,'" *Social Science & Medicine* 63 (2006): 843–45.

2. C. Smith and M. L. Denton, *Soul Searching: The Religious and Spiritual Lives of American Teenagers* (New York: Oxford University Press, 2005), 175.

3. K. I. Pargament, "The Psychology of Religion and Spirituality? Yes and No," *International Journal for the Psychology of Religion* 9 (1999): 3–16.

4. H. G. Koenig, "An 83-Year-Old Woman with Chronic Illness and Strong Religious Beliefs," *Journal of the American Medical Association* 288, no. 4 (2002): 487–93.

5. B. Lo, T. Quill, and J. Tulsky, "Discussing Palliative Care with Patients," *Annals of Internal Medicine* 130 (1999): 744–49.

6. C. M. Puchalski and A. L. Romer, "Taking a Spiritual History Allows Clinicians to Understand Patients More Fully," *Journal of Palliative Medicine* 3 (2000): 129–37.

7. H. G. Koenig, L. Bearon, and R. Dayringer, "Physician Perspectives on the Role of Religion in the Physician–Older Patient Relationship," *Journal of Family Practice* 28 (1989): 441–48.

8. If the HP communicates to the patient that he or she will be praying for the patient, it is always important that permission be requested from the patient to do this. If the HP does not tell the patient that he or she is doing this, then, in my opinion, no permission from the patient is necessary.

9. R. P. Sloan, E. Bagiella, L. VandeCreek, M. Hover, C. Casalone, T. J. Hirsch, Y. Hasan, and R. Kreger, "Should Physicians Prescribe Religious Activities?" *New England Journal of Medicine* 342 (2000): 1913–16.

10. Koenig, Bearon, and Dayringer, "Physician Perspectives on the Role of Religion in the Physician–Older Patient Relationship."

11. H. G. Koenig, M. Smiley, and J. Gonzales, *Religion, Health, and Aging* (Westport, CT: Greenwood Press, 1988).

12. D. E. King and B. Bushwick, "Beliefs and Attitudes of Hospital Inpatients about Faith Healing and Prayer," *Journal of Family Practice* 39 (1994): 349–52; L. C. Kaldjian, J. F. Jekel, and G. Friedland, "End-of-Life Decisions in HIV-Positive Patients: The Role of Spiritual Beliefs," *AIDS* 12, no. 1 (1998): 103–7; O. Oyama and H. G. Koenig, "Religious Beliefs and Practices in Family Medicine," *Archives of Family Medicine* 7 (1998): 431–35; C. D. MacLean, B. Susi, N. Phifer, L. Schultz, D. Bynum, M. Franco, A. Klioze, M. Monroe, J. Garrett, and S. Cykert, "Patient Preference for Physician Discussion and Practice of Spirituality," *Journal of General Internal Medicine* 18 (2003): 38–43.

13. Yankelovich Parners, Inc., for *Time*/CNN, June 1996.

14. MacLean et al., *Journal of General Internal Medicine.*

15. Koenig, Bearon, and Dayringer, "Physician Perspectives on the Role of Religion in the Physician–Older Patient Relationship."

16. J. T. Chibnall and C. A. Brooks, "Religion in the Clinic: The Role of Physician Beliefs," *Southern Medical Journal* 94 (2001): 374–79.

17. T. F. Dagi, "Prayer, Piety, and Professional Propriety: Limits on Religious Expression on Hospitals," *Journal of Clinical Ethics* 6 (1995): 274–79.

18. F. A. Curlin, M. H. Chin, S. A. Sellergren, C. J. Roach, and J. D. Lantos, "The Association of Physicians' Religious Characteristics with Their Attitudes and Self-Reported Behaviors Regarding Religion and Spirituality in the Clinical Encounter," *Medical Care* 44 (2006): 446–53.

19. Sloan et al., "Should Physicians Prescribe Religious Activities?"

20. W. E. Hale and R. G. Bennett, *Building Healthy Communities through Medical-Religious Partnerships* (Baltimore: Johns Hopkins University Press,

2000); L. J. Medvene, J. V. Wescott, A. Huckstadt, et al., "Promoting Signing of Advance Directives in Faith Communities," *Journal of General Internal Medicine* 18, no. 11 (2003): 914–20; G. Corbie-Smith, A. S. Ammerman, M. L. Katz, et al., "Trust, Benefit, Satisfaction, and Burden: A Randomized Controlled Trial to Reduce Cancer Risk through African-American Churches," *Journal of General Internal Medicine* 18, no. 7 (2003): 531–41; C. Hoyo, L. Reid, J. Hatch, et al., "Program Prioritization to Control Chronic Diseases in African-American Faith-Based Communities," *Journal of the National Medical Association* 96, no. 4 (2004): 524–32; L. R. Yanek, D. M. Becker, T. F. Moy, J. Gittelsohn, and D. M. Koffman, "Project Joy: Faith Based Cardiovascular Health Promotion for African American Women," *Public Health Reports* 116, supp. 1 (2001): 68–81.

21. See Web site, http://www.aoa.dhhs.gov/aoa/stats/AgePop2050.html.

22. E. L. Schneider, "Aging in the Third Millennium," *Science* 283 (1999): 796–97.

23. V. B. Carson and H. G. Koenig, *Parish Nursing: Stories of Service and Care* (Philadelphia, PA: Templeton Foundation Press, 2002).

CHAPTER 3: *WHEN* TO INCLUDE SPIRITUALITY

1. N. H. Cassem, H. A. Wishnie, and T. P. Hackett, "How Coronary Patients Respond to Last Rites," *Postgraduate Medicine* 45, no. 3 (1969): 147–52.

2. H. Benson and M. Stark, *Timeless Healing: The Power and Biology of Belief* (New York: Simon & Schuster, 1996).

3. B. D. Feldstein, "Toward Meaning," *Journal of the American Medical Association* 286 (2001): 1291–92.

4. T. F. Dagi, "Prayer, Piety, and Professional Propriety: Limits on Religious Expression in Hospitals," *Journal of Clinical Ethics* 6 (1995): 274–79.

5. S. G. Post, C. Puchalski, and D. Larson, "Physicians and Patient Spirituality: Professional Boundaries, Competency, and Ethics," *Annals of Internal Medicine* 132 (2000): 578–83.

CHAPTER 4: *WHAT* MIGHT RESULT?

1. Most established traditional religious belief systems present a positive worldview, even some of those that on the surface don't appear to do so (such as fundamentalist systems that focus on sin, judgment, and retribution, and have rules that are harsh, rigid, and inflexible). These systems offer structure and simple guidelines on how to obtain relief through religious solutions and are usually quite sympathetic to sickness and adversity (although not always).

2. L. R. Propst, R. Ostrom, P. Watkins, T. Dean, and D. Mashburn,

"Comparative Efficacy of Religious and Nonreligious Cognitive-Behavior Therapy for the Treatment of Clinical Depression in Religious Individuals," *Journal of Consulting and Clinical Psychology* 60 (1992): 94–103; M. Z. Azhar, S. L.Varma, and A. S. Dharap, "Religious Psychotherapy in Anxiety Disorder Patients," *Acta Psychiatrica Scandinavica* 90 (1994): 1–3; S. M. Razali, C. I. Hasanah, K. Aminah, and M. Subramaniam, "Religious-Sociocultural Psychotherapy in Patients with Anxiety and Depression," *Australian & New Zealand Journal of Psychiatry* 32 (1998): 867–72.

3. J. L. Kristeller, M. Rhodes, L. D. Cripe, and V. Sheets, "Oncologist Assisted Spiritual Intervention Study (OASIS): Patient Acceptability and Initial Evidence of Effects," *International Journal of Psychiatry in Medicine* 35 (2005): 329–47.

4. W. Osler, "The Faith That Heals," *The British Medical Journal* (1910): 1470–72.

5. D. G. Safran, D. A. Taira, W. H. Rogers, M. Kosinski, J. E. Ware, and A. R. Tarlov, "Linking Primary Care Performance to Outcomes of Care," *Journal of Family Practice* 47, no. 3 (1998): 213–20.

6. D. H. Thom, K. M. Ribisl, A. L. Stewart, and D. A. Luke, "Further Validation and Reliability Testing of the Trust in Physician Scale: The Stanford Trust Study Physicians," *Medical Care* 37, no. 5 (1999): 510–17.

7. H. G. Koenig, M. E. McCollough, and D. B. Larson, "Disease Prevention, Disease Detection, and Treatment Compliance," in *Handbook of Religion and Health* (New York: Oxford University Press, 2001), 397–408.

8. H. G. Koenig, F. Shelp, V. Goli, H. J. Cohen, and D. G. Blazer, "Survival and Healthcare Utilization in Elderly Medical Inpatients with Major Depression," *Journal of the American Geriatrics Society* 37 (1989): 599–606.

9. J. K. Kiecolt-Glaser, P. T. Marucha, W. B. Malarkey, A. M. Mercado, and R. Glaser, "Slowing of Wound Healing by Psychological Stress," *Lancet* 346, no. 8984 (1996): 1194–96.

10. H. Benson and M. Stark, *Timeless Healing: The Power and Biology of Belief* (New York: Simon & Schuster, 1996).

11. Kristeller, Rhodes, Cripe, and Sheets, "Oncologist Assisted Spiritual Intervention Study (OASIS): Patient Acceptability and Initial Evidence of Effects."

CHAPTER 5: BOUNDARIES AND BARRIERS

1. E. Pelligrino, "Toward a Reconstruction of Medical Morality: The Primacy of the Act of Profession and the Fact of Illness," *Journal of Medicine and Philosophy* 4 (1979): 32–56.

2. J. Forster, "Retake Your Hippocratic Oath," *Medical Economics*, January 10, 2000.

3. A. M. Butler, "Hippocratic Oath," *New England Journal of Medicine* 278 (1968): 48–49.

4. Translated by Harry Friedenwald, *Bulletin of the Johns Hopkins Hospital* 28 (1917): 260–61.

5. M. H. Spero, "Countertransference in Religious Therapists of Religious Patients," *American Journal of Psychotherapy* 35 (1981): 565–75.

6. M. R. Ellis, D. C. Vinson, and B. Ewigman, "Addressing Spiritual Concerns of Patients: Family Physicians' Attitudes and Practices," *Journal of Family Practice* 48 (1999): 105–9; F. A. Curlin, M. H. Chin, S. A. Sellergren, C. J. Roach, and J. D. Lantos, "The Association of Physicians' Religious Characteristics with Their Attitudes and Self-Reported Behaviors Regarding Religion and Spirituality in the Clinical Encounter," *Medical Care* 44 (2006): 446–53.

7. H. G. Koenig, M. Hover, L. B. Bearon, and J. L. Travis, "Religious Perspectives of Doctors, Nurses, Patients and Families: Some Interesting Differences," *Journal of Pastoral Care* 45 (1991): 254–67.

8. K. G. Barnett and A. H. Fortin, "Spirituality and Medicine: A Workshop for Medical Students and Residents," *Journal of General Internal Medicine* 21, no. 5 (2006): 481–85.

9. Ellis, Vinson, and Ewigman, "Addressing Spiritual Concerns of Patients: Family Physicians' Attitudes and Practices."

10. J. T. Chibnall and C. A. Brooks, "Religion in the Clinic: The Role of Physician Beliefs," *Southern Medical Journal* 94 (2001): 374–79.

11. Curlin et al., "The Association of Physicians' Religious Characteristics with Their Attitudes and Self-Reported Behaviors Regarding Religion and Spirituality in the Clinical Encounter."

12. H. P. Chalfant, P. L. Heller, A. Roberts, D. Briones, S. Aquirre-Hochbaum, and W. Farr, "The Clergy as a Resource for Those Encountering Psychological Distress," *Review of Religious Research* 31 (1990): 305–13; D. B. Larson, A. A. Hohmann, L. G. Kessler, K. G. Meador, J. H. Boyd, and E. McSherry, "The Couch and the Cloth: The Need for Linkage," *Hospital and Community Psychiatry* 39 (1988): 1064–69.

13. Chibnall and Brooks, "Religion in the Clinic: The Role of Physician Beliefs."

14. Curlin et al., "The Association of Physicians' Religious Characteristics with Their Attitudes and Self-Reported Behaviors Regarding Religion and Spirituality in the Clinical Encounter."

15. Chibnall and Brooks, "Religion in the Clinic: The Role of Physician Beliefs."

16. H. G. Koenig, L. Bearon, and R. Dayringer, "Physician Perspectives on the Role of Religion in the Physician–Older Patient Relationship," *Journal of Family Practice* 28 (1989): 441–48.

17. Chibnall and Brooks, "Religion in the Clinic: The Role of Physician Beliefs."

18. M. H. Monroe, D. Bynum, B. Susi, N. Phifer, L. Schultz, M. Franco, C. D. MacLean, S. Cykert, and J. Garrett, *Archives of Internal Medicine* 163 (2003): 2751–56.

19. Ellis, Vinson, and Ewigman, "Addressing Spiritual Concerns of Patients: Family Physicians' Attitudes and Practices."

20. Koenig, Bearon, and Dayringer, "Physician Perspectives on the Role of Religion in the Physician–Older Patient Relationship."

21. T. A. Maugans and W. C. Wadland, "Religion and Family Medicine: A Survey of Physicians and Patients," *Journal of Family Practice* 32 (1991): 210–13.

22. Curlin et al., "The Association of Physicians' Religious Characteristics with Their Attitudes and Self-Reported Behaviors Regarding Religion and Spirituality in the Clinical Encounter."

CHAPTER 6: WHEN RELIGION (OR SPIRITUALITY) IS HARMFUL

1. R. P. Sloan, E. Bagiella, and T. Powell, "Religion, Spirituality, and Medicine," *The Lancet* 353 (1999): 664–67.

2. R. P. Sloan, E. Bagiella, L. VandeCreek, M. Hover, C. Casalone, T. J. Hirsch, Y. Hasan, and R. Kreger, "Should Physicians Prescribe Religious Activities?" *New England Journal of Medicine* 342 (2000): 1913–16.

3. J. J. Exline, "Stumbling Blocks on the Religious Road: Fractured Relationships, Nagging Vices, and the Inner Struggle to Believe," *Psychological Inquiry* 13 (2002): 182–89.

4. C. Spence, T. S. Danielson, and W. M. Kaunitz, "The Faith Assembly: A Study of Perinatal and Maternal Mortality," *Indiana Medicine* (March 1984): 180–83.

5. M. A. Conyn–Van Spaendonck, H. E. de Melker, F. Abbink, N. Elzinga–Gholizadea, T. G. Kimman, and T. van Loon, "Immunity to Poliomyelitis in the Netherlands," *American Journal of Epidemiology* 153, no. 3 (2001): 207–14.

6. "Outbreaks of Rubella among the Amish—United States, 1991," *Morbidity and Mortality Weekly Report* 40, no. 16 (1991): 264–65.

7. P. Etkind, S. M. Lett, P. D. MacDonald, E. Silva, and J. Peppe, "Pertussis Outbreaks in Groups Claiming Religious Exemptions to Vaccinations," *American Journal of Diseases of Children* 146 (1992): 173–76.

8. D. V. Rodgers, J. S. Gindler, W. L. Atkinson, and L. E. Markowitz, "High Attack Rates and Case Fatality during a Measles Outbreak in Groups with Religious Exemption to Vaccination," *Pediatric Infectious Disease Journal* 12 (1993): 288–92.

9. S. B. Omer, W. K. Pan, N. A. Halsey, S. Stokley, L. H. Moulton, A. M. Navar, M. Pierce, and D. A. Salmon, "Nonmedical Exemptions to School Immunization Requirements: Secular Trends and Association of State Policies with Pertussis Incidence," *Journal of the American Medical Association* 296, no. 14 (2006): 1757–63.

10. D. V. Coakley and G. W. McKenna, "Safety of Faith Healing," *Lancet*, February 22, 1986, 444; D. M. Smith, "Safety of Faith Healing," *Lancet*, March 15, 1986, 621.

11. S. Asser and R. Swan, "Child Fatalities from Religion-Motivated Medical Neglect," *Pediatrics* 101 (1998): 625–29.

12. H. G. Koenig, M. E. McCollough, and D. B. Larson, *Handbook of Religion and Health* (New York: Oxford University Press, 2001), 63–71.

13. K. I. Pargament, H. G. Koenig, N. Tarakeshwar, and J. Hahn, "Religious Struggle as a Predictor of Mortality among Medically Ill Elderly Patients: A Two-Year Longitudinal Study," *Archives of Internal Medicine* 161 (2001): 1881–85.

14. J. L. Kristeller, M. Rhodes, L. D. Cripe, and V. Sheets, "Oncologist Assisted Spiritual Intervention Study (OASIS): Patient Acceptability and Initial Evidence of Effects," *International Journal of Psychiatry in Medicine* 35 (2005): 329–47.

15. R. P. Sloan, E. Bagiella, and T. Powell, "Religion, Spirituality, and Medicine," 666.

16. Pargament, Koenig, Tarakeshwar, and Hahn, "Religious Struggle as a Predictor of Mortality among Medically Ill Elderly Patients: A Two-Year Longitudinal Study."

CHAPTER 7: CHAPLAINS AND PASTORAL CARE

1. APC Web site, http://www.professionalchaplains.org/uploadedFiles/pdf/common-standards-professional-chaplaincy.pdf.

2. APC Web site, http://www.professionalchaplains.org/.

3. NACC Web site, http://www.nacc.org/aboutnacc/default.asp.

4. NAJC Web site, http://www.najc.org/main/index.htm.

5. ACPE Web site, http://www.acpe.edu/.

6. "Guidelines for the Chaplain's Role in Health Care Ethics," APC Web site, http://www.professionalchaplains.org/index.aspx?id=222.

7. "Evaluating Your Spiritual Assessment Process," *Joint Commission: The Source* 3, no. 2 (2005): 6–7; see http://www.professionalchaplains.org/uploadedFiles/pdf/JCAHO-evaluating-your-spiritual-assessment-process.pdf.

8. K. J. Flannelly, K. Galek, and G. F. Handzo, "To What Extent Are the Spiritual Needs of Hospital Patients Being Met?" *International Journal of Psychiatry in Medicine* 35, no. 3 (2005): 319–23.

9. G. Fitchett, *The 7 x 7 Model for Spiritual Assessment*, cassette (Schaumberg, IL: Association of Professional Chaplains, 1995).

10. L. VandeCreek, and A. M. Lucas, *The Discipline for Pastoral Care Giving: Foundations for Outcome Oriented Chaplaincy* (Binghamton, NY: Haworth Pastoral Press, 2001).

11. G. Berg. "The Use of Computer as a Tool for Assessment and Research in Pastoral Care," *Journal of Health Care Chaplaincy* 6 (1994): 11–25.

12. See the chaplain code of ethics at the Association of Professional Chaplains Web site, http://www.professionalchaplains.org/uploadedFiles/pdf/code_of_ethics_2003.pdf.

13. C. G. Sharp, "The Use of Chaplaincy in the Neonatal Intensive Care Unit," *Southern Medical Journal* 84, no. 12 (1991): 1482–86.

14. Association of Professional Chaplains "Code of Ethics": see Web site http://www.professionalchaplains.org/index.aspx?id=85&TierSlicer1_TSMen uTargetID=85&TierSlicer1_

15. Barna Research Group, "Unchurched," see http://www.barna.org/FlexPage.aspx?Page=Topic&TopicID=38.

16. See http://www.aapc.org/.

17. See http://www.aapc.org/history.htm.

CHAPTER 8: SPIRITUALITY IN NURSING CARE

1. V. B. Carson and H. G. Koenig, *Spiritual Dimensions of Nursing*, 2nd ed. (not yet published); M. E. O'Brien, *Spirituality in Nursing: Standing on Holy Ground* (Boston: Jones & Bartlett, 1999); J. A. Shelly and A. B. Miller, *Called to Care: A Christian Worldview of Nursing*, 2nd ed. (Downers Grove, IL: Intervarsity, 2006); B. S. Barnum, *Spirituality in Nursing: From Traditional to New Age*, 2nd ed. (New York: Springer, 2003).

2. V. B. Carson, *Spiritual Dimensions of Nursing Practice* (St. Louis, MO: Saunders, 1989).

3. M. Colliton, "The Spiritual Dimension of Nursing," in *Clinical Nursing*, 4th ed., ed. I. Beland and J. Y. Passos (New York: Macmillan, 1981).

4. J. Stallwood and R. Stoll, "Spiritual Dimension of Nursing Practice," in *Clinical Nursing*, 3rd ed., ed. I. Beland and J. Y. Passos (New York: Macmillan, 1975).

5. K. Wright, "Professional, Ethical, and Legal Implications for Spiritual Care in Nursing," *Image: Journal of Nursing Scholarship* 30 (1998): 81–83.

6. A. Narayanasamy, "Learning Spiritual Dimensions of Care from a Historical Perspective," *Nurse Education Today* 19 (1999): 386–95; E. J. Taylor, *Spiritual Care* (Englewood Cliffs, NJ: Prentice Hall, 2002).

7. D. Grant, "Spiritual Interventions: How, When, and Why Nurses Use Them," *Holistic Nursing Practice* 18, no. 1 (2004): 36–41.

8. A. Narayanasamy, "Nurses' Awareness and Educational Preparation in Meeting Their Patients' Spiritual Needs," *Nurse Education Today* 13 (1993): 196–201.

9. S. Stranahan, "Spiritual Perception, Attitudes about Spiritual Care, and Spiritual Care Practices among Nurse Practitioners," *Western Journal of Nursing Research* 23, no. 1 (2001): 90–104.

10. S. L. Hubbell, E. K. Woodard, D. J. Barksdale-Brown, and J. S. Parker, "Spiritual Care Practices of Nurse Practitioners in Federally Designated Nonmetropolitan Areas of North Carolina," *Journal of the American Academy of Nurse Practitioners* 18, no. 8 (2006): 379–85.

11. C. Piles, "Providing Spiritual Care," *Nurse Educator* 16, no. 1 (1990): 36–41.

12. L. Pullen, I. Tuck, and K. Mix, "Mental Health Nurses' Spiritual Perspectives," *Journal of Holistic Nursing* 14, no. 2 (1996): 85–97.

13. C. Lemmer, "Teaching the Spiritual Dimension of Care: A Survey of U.S. Baccalaureate Nursing Programs," *Journal of Nursing Education* 42 (2002): 482–90; J. Olson, P. Paul, L. Douglass, M. Clark, J. Simington, and N. Goddard, "Addressing the Spiritual Dimension in Canadian Undergraduate Nursing Education," *Canadian Journal of Nursing Research* 35 (2003): 94–107; E. J. Taylor, "What Have We Learned from Spiritual Care Research?" *Journal of Christian Nursing* 22 (2005): 22–29.

14. Lemmer, "Teaching the Spiritual Dimension of Care: A Survey of U.S. Baccalaureate Nursing Programs."

15. Olson et al., "Addressing the Spiritual Dimension in Canadian Undergraduate Nursing Education."

16. K. Sodestrom and I. Martinson, "Patients' Spiritual Coping Strategies: A Study of Nurse and Patient Perspectives," *Oncology Nursing Forum* 14, no. 2 (1987): 41–46.

17. H. G. Koenig, M. Hover, L. B. Bearon, and J. L. Travis, "Religious Perspectives of Doctors, Nurses, Patients and Families: Some Interesting Differences," *Journal of Pastoral Care* 45 (1991): 254–67.

18. K. J. Flannelly, A. J. Weaver, and G. F. Handzo, "A Three-Year Study of Chaplains' Professional Activities at Memorial Sloan-Kettering Cancer Center in New York City," *Psycho-Oncology* 12, no. 8 (2003): 760–68.

CHAPTER 9: SPIRITUALITY IN SOCIAL WORK

1. North American Association of Christians in Social Work; see Web site, http://www.nacsw.org/index.shtml.

2. Society for Spirituality and Social Work; see Web site, http://ssw.asu.edu/spirituality/sssw/.

3. Canadian Society for Spirituality and Social Work; see Web site, http://people.stu.ca/~jcoates/cnssw/.

4. Center for Spirituality and Integral Social Work at The Catholic University of America; see Web site, http://csisw.cua.edu.

5. E. R. Canda, ed., *Spirituality in Social Work: New Directions* (Binghamton, NY: Haworth Pastoral Press, 1998); D. S. Becvar, *The Family, Spirituality, and Social Work* (Binghamton, NY: Haworth Press, 1998); E. R. Canda and L. D.

Furman, *Spiritual Diversity in Social Work Practice: The Heart of Helping* (New York: Free Press, 1999).

6. P. A. Gilligan, "It Isn't Discussed. Religion, Belief and Practice Teaching: Missing Components of Cultural Competence in Social Work Education," *Journal of Practice Teaching in Health and Social Work* 5, no. 1 (2003): 75–95; L. D. Furman, P. W. Benson, C. Grimwood, and E. Canda, "Religion and Spirituality in Social Work Education and Direct Practice at the Millennium: A Survey of UK Social Workers," *British Journal of Social Work* 34, no. 6 (2004): 767–92.

7. C. Stewart, G. F. Koeske, and R. D. Koeske, "Personal Religiosity and Spirituality Associated with Social Work Practitioners' Use of Religious-Based Intervention Practices," *Journal of Religion & Spirituality in Social Work* 25, no. 1 (2006): 69–85.

8. V. Murdock, "Guided by Ethics: Religion and Spirituality in Gerontological Social Work Practice," *Journal of Gerontological Social Work* 45, no. 1/2 (2005): 131–54.

9. M. J. Sheridan, "Predicting the Use of Spiritually-Derived Interventions in Social Work Practice: A Survey of Practitioners," *Journal of Religion & Spirituality in Social Work* 23, no. 4 (2004): 5–25.

10. D. R. Hodge, "Spiritual Lifemaps: A Client-Centered Pictorial Instrument for Spiritual Assessment, Planning, and Intervention," *Social Work* 50, no. 1 (2005): 77–87.

CHAPTER 10: SPIRITUALITY IN REHABILITATION

1. Christian Physical Therapists International; see Web site, http://www.cpti.org/.

2. International Occupational Therapists for Christ, Inc.; see Web site, http://www.otforchrist.org.

3. Multicultural Occupational Therapy Networking Groups; see American Association of Occupational Therapy Web site, http://www.aota.org/featured/area2/links/link26.asp.

4. See Web site, http://www.cpti.org/about.html.

5. E. Oakley, G. Katz, K. Sauer, and B. Dent, "Physical Therapists Perception on Spirituality and Patient Care: Beliefs, Practices and Perceived Barriers," *Journal of the American Physical Therapy Association,* June 30–July 3, 2004, www.apta.org/am/abstracts/pt2004/abstractspt2004.cfm?pubNo=PO-RR-113-TH.

6. J. C. Pitts, "Perceptions of Physical Therapy Faculty on the Inclusion of Spirituality in Physical Therapy Education" (doctoral dissertation, Andrews University, 2005), 180.

7. Canadian Association of Occupational Therapists, *Occupational Therapy Guidelines for Client-Centred Practice* (Author: Toronto, 1991), 3.

8. J. Blain and E. Townsend, "Occupational Therapy Guidelines for Client-Centred Practice: Impact Study Findings," *Canadian Journal of Occupational Therapy* 60, no. 5 (1993): 271–85; D. Engquist, M. Short–DeGraff, J. Gliner, and K. Oltjenbruns, "Occupational Therapists' Beliefs and Practices with Regard to Spirituality and Therapy," *American Journal of Occupational Therapy* 51, no. 3 (1997): 173–80.

9. J. E. Farrar, "Addressing Spirituality and Religious Life in Occupational Therapy Practice," *Physical & Occupational Therapy in Geriatrics* 18, no. 4 (2001): 65–85.

10. E. Taylor, J. E. Mitchell, S. Kenan, and R. Tacker, "Attitudes of Occupational Therapists toward Spirituality in Practice," *American Journal of Occupational Therapy* 54, no. 4 (2000): 421–28.

11. M. S. Rosenfeld, "Spiritual Agent Modalities for Occupational Therapy Practice," *OT Practice*, January 17–21, 2000.

CHAPTER 11: SPIRITUALITY IN MENTAL HEALTH CARE

1. H. G. Koenig, *Handbook of Religion and Mental Health* (San Diego: Academic Press, 1998).

2. E. P. Shafranske, *Religion and the Clinical Practice of Psychology* (Washington, DC: American Psychological Association, 1996); P. S. Richards and A. E. Bergin, *Handbook of Psychotherapy and Religious Diversity* (Washington, DC: American Psychological Association, 2000).

3. R. J. Wicks, R. D. Parsons, and D. Capps, *Clinical Handbook of Pastoral Care* (New York: Paulist Press, 2003).

4. S. Freud, "Future of an Illusion," in *Standard Edition of the Complete Psychological Works of Sigmund Freud*, ed. and trans. J. Strachey (1927; London: Hogarth Press, 1962), 43; A. Ellis, "Psychotherapy and Atheistic Values: A Response to A. E. Bergin's 'Psychotherapy and Religious Values,'" *Journal of Consulting and Clinical Psychology* 48 (1980): 635–39.

5. A. E. Bergin and J. P. Jensen, "Religiosity and Psychotherapists: A National Survey," *Psychotherapy* 27 (1990): 3–7.

6. H. G. Koenig, M. Hover, L. B. Bearon, and J. L. Travis, "Religious Perspectives of Doctors, Nurses, Patients and Families: Some Interesting Differences," *Journal of Pastoral Care* 45 (1991): 254–67.

7. A. J. Weaver, "Has There Been a Failure to Prepare and Support Parish-Based Clergy in Their Role as Front-Line Community Mental Health Workers? A Review," *Journal of Pastoral Care* 49 (1995): 129–49; H. G. Koenig, *Faith and Mental Health: Religious Resources for Healing* (Philadelphia, PA: Templeton Foundation Press, 2005), 173–74.

8. D. B. Larson, A. A. Hohmann, L. G. Kessler, K. G. Meador, J. H. Boyd, and E. McSherry, "The Couch and the Cloth: The Need for Linkage," *Hospital and Community Psychiatry* 39 (1988): 1064–69.

9. Koenig, *Faith and Mental Health: Religious Resources for Healing*, 43–112.

10. Ibid., 145–48.

11. Ibid., 113–32.

12. H. G. Koenig, "Schizophrenia and Other Psychotic Disorders," in *Religion and Psychiatric Disorders in DSM-V*, ed. F. Lu and J. Peteet (Washington, DC: American Psychiatric Publishing, 2008).

13. R. Thara and W. W. Eaton, "Outcome of Schizophrenia: The Madras Longitudinal Study," *Australian and New Zealand J Psychiatry* 30 (1996): 516–22; S. Doering, E. Muller, W. Kopcke, et al., "Predictors of Relapse and Rehospitalisation in Schizophrenia and Schizoaffective Disorder," *Schizophrenia Bulletin* 24 (1998): 87–98.

14. D. Lukoff, "The Diagnosis of Mystical Experiences with Psychotic Features," *Journal of Transpersonal Psychology* 17, no. 2 (1985): 155–81; J. M. Pierre, "Faith or Delusion: At the Crossroads of Religion and Psychosis," *Journal of Psychiatric Practice* 7, no. 3 (2001): 163–72.

15. M. H. Spero, "Countertransference in Religious Therapists of Religious Patients," *American Journal of Psychotherapy* 35 (1981): 565–75.

16. A. Fontana and R. Rosenheck, "Trauma, Change in Strength of Religious Faith, and Mental Health Service Use among Veterans Treated for PTSD," *Journal of Nervous & Mental Disease* 192 (2004): 579-584.

17. M. Bobgan and D. Bobgan, *Prophets of Psychoheresy I* (Santa Barbara: EastGate Publishers, 1989); M. Bobgan and D. Bobgan, *Prophets of Psychoheresy II* (Santa Barbara: EastGate Publishers, 1990).

18. J. Adams, *Competent to Counsel* (Grand Rapids, MI: Zondervan, 1986).

19. D. Biebel and H. G. Koenig, *New Light on Depression* (Grand Rapids, MI: Zondervan, 2004).

CHAPTER 12: A MODEL COURSE CURRICULUM

1. Spirituality and Medicine Interest Group at the Medical University of South Carolina, see Web site http://www.musc.edu/dfm/Spirituality/Spirituality.htm; and, The George Washington Institute for Spirituality and Health (GWISH), see Web site, http://www.gwish.org/.

2. H. G. Koenig, "Religion and Medicine I: Historical Background and Reasons for Separation," *International Journal of Psychiatry in Medicine* 30 (2000): 385–98.

3. H. G. Koenig, L. K. George, and B. L. Peterson, "Religiosity and Remission of Depression in Medically Ill Older Patients," *American Journal of Psychiatry* 155, no. 4 (1998): 536–42; H. G. Koenig, "Religion and Depression in Older Medical Inpatients," *American Journal of Geriatric Psychiatry* 15 (2007)): (April), in press ; H. G. Koenig, "Religion and Remission of Depression in Medical Inpatients with Heart Failure/Pulmonary Disease," *Journal of Nervous and Mental Disease* 195 (2007): (May/June), in press.

4. W. J. Strawbridge, R. D. Cohen, S. J. Shema, and G. A. Kaplan, "Frequent Attendance at Religious Services and Mortality over 28 Years," *American Journal of Public Health* 87 (1997): 957–61; S. K. Lutgendorf, D. Russell, P. Ullrich, T. B. Harris, and R. Wallace, "Religious Participation, Interleukin-6, and Mortality in Older Adults," *Health Psychology* 23, no. 5 (2004): 465–75.

5. R. P. Sloan, E. Bagiella, and T. Powell, "Religion, Spirituality, and Medicine," *The Lancet* 353 (1999): 664–67; H. G. Koenig, E. Idler, S. Kasl, J. Hays, L. K. George, M. Musick, D. B. Larson, T. Collins, and H. Benson, "Religion, Spirituality, and Medicine: A Rebuttal to Skeptics," *International Journal of Psychiatry in Medicine* 29 (1999): 123–31; P. S. Mueller, D. J. Plevak, and T. A. Rummans, "Religious Involvement, Spirituality, and Medicine: Implications for Clinical Practice," *Mayo Clinic Proceedings* 76, no. 12 (2001): 1225–35.

6. H. G. Koenig, "An 83-Year-Old Woman with Chronic Illness and Strong Religious Beliefs," *Journal of the American Medical Association* 288, no. 4 (2002): 487–93.

7. H. G. Koenig, "Taking a Spiritual History," *Journal of the American Medical Association* 291 (2004): 2881.

8. H. G. Koenig, "Religion, Spirituality and Medicine: Research Findings and Implications for Clinical Practice," *Southern Medical Journal* 97 (2004): 1194–1200.

9. C. B. Cohen, S. E. Wheeler, and D. A. Scott, "Walking a Fine Line: Physician Inquiries into Patients' Religious and Spiritual Beliefs," *Hastings Center Report* (September/October 2001): 29–39.

10. J. L. Kristeller, M. Rhodes, L. D. Cripe, and V. Sheets, "Oncologist Assisted Spiritual Intervention Study (OASIS): Patient Acceptability and Initial Evidence of Effects," *International Journal of Psychiatry in Medicine* 35 (2005): 329–47.

11. S. G. Post, C. Puchalski, and D. Larson, "Physicians and Patient Spirituality: Professional Boundaries, Competency, and Ethics," *Annals of Internal Medicine* 132 (2000): 578–83.

12 I. C. Lupu and R. W. Tuttle, "Freedom from Religion Foundation, Inc. (and others) vs. R. James Nicholson, Secretary of the Department of Veterans Affairs (and others)," *The Roundtable on Religion and Social Welfare Policy*, May 30, 2006 (http://www.religionandsocialpolicy.org/legal/legal_update_display.cfm?id=48), with January 16, 2007 update, "Federal Court Strikes Down Challenge to VA Chaplaincy Program" (http://www.religionandsocialpolicy.org/news/article.cfm?id=5890)

13. R. P. Sloan, E. Bagiella, L. VandeCreek, M. Hover, C. Casalone, T. J. Hirsch, Y. Hasan, and R. Kreger, "Should Physicians Prescribe Religious Activities?" *New England Journal of Medicine* 342 (2000): 1913–16.

14. H. G. Koenig, "Religion and Medicine: Letter in Response to 'Should

Physicians Prescribe Religious Activities?'" *New England Journal of Medicine* 343 (2000): 1339.

15. V. B. Carson and H. G. Koenig, *Spiritual Caregiving for the Health Professional*, 2nd ed. (St. Louis, MO: Elsevier, 2007); M. E. O'Brien, *Spirituality in Nursing: Standing on Holy Ground* (Boston: Jones & Bartlett, 1999); B. S. Barnum, *Spirituality in Nursing: From Traditional to New Age*, 2nd ed. (New York: Springer, 2003).

16. A. Fontana and R. Rosenheck, "Trauma, Change in Strength of Religious Faith, and Mental Health Service Use among Veterans Treated for PTSD," *Journal of Nervous & Mental Disease* 192 (2004): 579-584.

17. S. S. Doe, "Spirituality-Based Social Work Values for Empowering Human Service Organizations," *Journal of Religion & Spirituality in Social Work* 23, no. 3 (2004): 45–65; L. J. Praglin, "Spirituality, Religion, and Social Work: An Effort towards Interdisciplinary Conversation," *Journal of Religion & Spirituality in Social Work* 23, no. 4 (2004): 67–84; D. R. Hodge, "Developing a Spiritual Assessment Toolbox: A Discussion of the Strengths and Limitations of Five Different Assessment Methods," *Health and Social Work* 30, no. 4 (2005): 314–23.

18. M. A. McColl, "Spirit, Occupation and Disability," *Canadian Journal of Occupational Therapy* 67, no. 4 (2000): 217–28; C. Coyne, "Addressing Spirituality Issues in Patient Interventions: A Patient's Belief Structure Can Play a Role in the Patient's Health and the Effectiveness of Interventions," *PT—Magazine of Physical Therapy* 13, no. 7 (2005): 38–44; D. Johnston and C. Mayers, "Spirituality: A Review of How Occupational Therapists Acknowledge, Assess and Meet Spiritual Needs," *British Journal of Occupational Therapy* 68, no. 9 (2005): 386–92.

CHAPTER 13: INFORMATION ON SPECIFIC RELIGIONS

1. V. B. Carson, "Spirituality, Religion and Health Care: Examining the Relationships," in *Spiritual Dimensions of Nursing*, 2nd ed., ed. V. B. Carson and H. G. Koenig, chaps. 3 and 4 (not yet published).

2. S. Wintz and E. Cooper, *Learning Module: Cultural and Spiritual Sensitivity: A Quick Guide to Cultures and Spiritual Traditions* (Schaumburg, IL: Association of Professional Chaplains, 2003); for the full text, see http://www.professionalchaplains.org/uploadedFiles/pdf/learning-cultural-sensitivity.pdf.

3. B. Johnson, R. Stark, et al., *American Piety in the 21st Century: The Baylor Religion Survey* (Waco, TX: Baylor Institute for Studies of Religion Department of Sociology, Baylor University, 2006).

4. Description of Judaism, http://www.religioustolerance.org/jud_desc.htm.

5. "Top 20 Religions in the USA," http://www.adherents.com/rel_USA.html#religions.

6. "Hindu-Americans," http://www-unix.oit.umass.edu/~efhayes/hindu. htm.

7. "Buddhist Beliefs Affecting Health Care," http://www.healthsystem. virginia.edu/internet/chaplaincy/buddhism.cfm.

8. "Voices of the Lao Community," http://ethnomed.org/voices/lao.html.

9. "Taoism (a.k.a. Daoism)," http://www.religioustolerance.org/taoism. htm.

10. "Native American Spirituality," http://www.religioustolerance.org/ nataspir.htm.

11. For more information, see http://www.religioustolerance.org/santeri. htm.

12. "Hispanic Health," http://www.spanishpronto.homestead.com/ HispanicHealth.html.

13. For more information, see http://www.religioustolerance.org/voodoo. htm.

CHAPTER 14: SUMMARY OF KEY POINTS

1. Speaking mainly to health professionals who are not professional healthcare chaplains.

INDEX